FAMILY MEDICAL GUIDE

Other Publications:

AMERICAN COUNTRY

VOYAGE THROUGH THE UNIVERSE

THE THIRD REICH

THE TIME-LIFE GARDENER'S GUIDE

MYSTERIES OF THE UNKNOWN

TIME FRAME

FIX IT YOURSELF

FITNESS, HEALTH & NUTRITION

SUCCESSFUL PARENTING

HEALTHY HOME COOKING

UNDERSTANDING COMPUTERS

LIBRARY OF NATIONS

THE ENCHANTED WORLD

THE KODAK LIBRARY OF CREATIVE PHOTOGRAPHY

GREAT MEALS IN MINUTES

THE CIVIL WAR

PLANET EARTH

COLLECTOR'S LIBRARY OF THE CIVIL WAR

THE EPIC OF FLIGHT

THE GOOD COOK

WORLD WAR II

HOME REPAIR AND IMPROVEMENT

THE OLD WEST

FAMILY
MEDICAL GUIDE

TIME-LIFE BOOKS
ALEXANDRIA, VIRGINIA

Fix It Yourself was produced by
ST. REMY PRESS

MANAGING EDITOR	Kenneth Winchester
MANAGING ART DIRECTOR	Pierre Léveillé

Staff for *Family Medical Guide*

Series Editor	Brian Parsons
Series Assistant Editor	Kent J. Farrell
Editor	Adena Franz
Series Art Director	Diane Denoncourt
Art Director	Solange Laberge Pelland
Research Editor	Naomi Fukuyama
Designers	Lousnak Abdalian, Robert Galarneau, Julie Léger
Contributing Writers	Beth Asher, Janice P. Clarini, Linda Jarosiewicz, Andrea Jonhston, J. Sorrentino
Contributing Illustrators	Gérard Mariscalchi, Jacques Proulx
Cover	Robert Monté
Index	Christine M. Jacobs
Administrator	Denise Rainville
Accounting Manager	Natalie Watanabe
Production Manager	Michelle Turbide
Coordinator	Dominique Gagné
Systems Coordinator	Jean-Luc Roy
Studio Director	Maryo Proulx

Time-Life Books Inc. is a wholly owned subsidiary of
THE TIME INC. BOOK COMPANY

President and Chief Executive Officer	Kelso F. Sutton
President, Time Inc. Books Direct	Christopher T. Linen

TIME-LIFE BOOKS INC.

EDITOR	George Constable
Director of Design	Louis Klein
Director of Editorial Resources	Phyllis K. Wise
Director of Photography and Research	John Conrad Weiser
PRESIDENT	John M. Fahey Jr.
Senior Vice Presidents	Robert M. DeSena, Paul R. Stewart, Curtis G. Viebranz, Joseph J. Ward
Vice Presidents	Stephen L. Bair, Bonita L. Boezeman, Mary P. Donohoe, Stephen L. Goldstein, Juanita T. James, Andrew P. Kaplan, Trevor Lunn, Susan J. Maruyama, Robert H. Smith
New Product Development	Trevor Lunn, Donia Ann Steele
Supervisor of Quality Control	James King
PUBLISHER	Joseph J. Ward

Editorial Operations

Production	Celia Beattie
Library	Louise D. Forstall
Correspondents	Elisabeth Kraemer-Singh (Bonn); Christina Lieberman (New York); Maria Vincenza Aloisi (Paris); Ann Natanson (Rome).

THE CONSULTANTS

Consulting editor **David L. Harrison** served as an editor for several Time-Life Books do-it-yourself series, including *Home Repair and Improvement, The Encyclopedia of Gardening* and *The Art of Sewing.*

Michael Castleman, former editor of *Medical SelfCare* magazine, is the author of several articles and books, including *Cold Cures*, on health care. He specializes in consumer health information.

Karen Honegger, R.N., is currently employed as a nursing coordinator at the Salvation Army Catherine Booth Hospital Centre in Montreal, Quebec.

Gail Kelsall, R.N., B.A. (N), a critical care nurse with years of experience in various settings, is a graduate of Winnipeg General Hospital. She is currently Head Nurse of the Intensive Care Unit, Queen Elizabeth Hospital, Montreal.

Francine Languedoc, M.D., is a family physician practicing in Montreal. She obtained her B.Sc. in microbiology and an M.D. at McGill University.

A. Earl Mgebroff, M.D., is a family physician in Yoakum, Texas and is Clinical Associate Professor of Family Practice at the University of Texas Health Science Center in San Antonio. He is a charter member of the American Academy of Family Physicians and is the author of *Healthy and Whole*, a preventive medicine guide for laypersons.

Caroline Miller served as an editor for the Time-Life *Fix-It-Yourself* series. She works as a freelance editor and has written a number of book outlines for projects for Time-Life.

M. Dudley Phillips, M.D., is a family physician and has practiced medicine in Darlington, Maryland, for 42 years.

Library of Congress Cataloging-in-Publication Data
Family Medical Guide
      p. cm. – (Fix it yourself)
    Includes index.
    ISBN 0-8094-7412-3 (trade).
    ISBN 0-8094-7413-1 (library).
    1. Medicine, Popular.
    I. Time-Life Books. II. Series.
    RC81.F239 1990
    616—dc20   90-10992
                             CIP

For information about any Time-Life book, please write:
Reader Information
Time-Life Customer Service
P.O. Box C-32068
Richmond, Virginia
23261-2068

© 1990 Time-Life Books Inc. All rights reserved.
No part of this book may be reproduced in any form or by any electronic or mechanical means, including information storage and retrieval devices or systems, without prior written permission from the publisher, except that brief passages may be quoted for reviews.
First printing. Printed in U.S.A.
Published simultaneously in Canada.
School and library distribution by Silver Burdett Company, Morristown, New Jersey.

TIME-LIFE is a trademark of Time Incorporated U.S.A.

CONTENTS

HOW TO USE THIS BOOK

Family Medical Guide is divided into three sections. The Emergency Guide on pages 8 to 29 provides information that can be lifesaving in the event you must deal with a family medical emergency at home. Take the time to study this section *before* you need the important information it contains.

The procedures section—the heart of the book—is a comprehensive approach to troubleshooting and handling as well as preventing family medical problems. Shown below are four sample pages from the chapter entitled Respiratory System with captions describing the various features of the book and how they work.

For example, if a family member is afflicted with a common cold, the Troubleshooting Guide on page 66 will direct you to the bottom of the same page for steps to take to help relieve the symptoms; you will be referred elsewhere in the chapter and the book for other specific procedures to follow such as relieving congestion *(page 67)* or a sore throat *(page 68)*. A family medical problem that may be a sign of a medical emergency is highlighted in the Troubleshooting Guide with a red cross (✚). Procedures on handling a family medical problem at home also include instructions on when you should consult a physician.

Introductory text
Describes the body system and common medical problems associated with it.

Anatomy illustrations
Locate and describe the key elements of the body system.

RESPIRATORY SYSTEM

Your respiratory system consists of the body organs that facilitate breathing—the complex and life-sustaining process by which your body takes oxygen, one of its basic fuels, from the air around you. The diagram on page 65 illustrates the major organs involved in the process. Air inhaled through the nose passes through a nasal cavity and enters the pharynx; air inhaled through the mouth passes over the tongue directly to the pharynx. The air then moves down through a branch-like system of passages into the bronchioles of each lung. At the tips of the bronchioles, tiny, sponge-like sacs conduct a complex exchange, taking oxygen out of the air in the lungs and passing it into the blood, and taking carbon dioxide out of the blood and passing it back into the air in the lungs. As the lungs contract, the waste air is pushed back up to be exhaled.

Because the respiratory system is an easy access route into the body for dust, fumes and microscopic organisms, its organs are prone to infections and ailments of many types. While some respiratory system infections such as the common cold are usually not serious, no respiratory system infection should ever be ignored. Any ailment affects the ability of the respiratory system to provide the body with the oxygen it needs; with improper treatment, an ailment can worsen and lead to secondary complications, especially in an infant or elderly person.

The Troubleshooting Guide *(page 66)* puts procedures for common respiratory ailments at your fingertips and refers you to pages 66 to 71 for more detailed information. Familiarize yourself with the procedures for treating a common cold *(page 66)*. Know how to stop a nosebleed *(page 69)*, how to evaluate and relieve a sore throat *(page 68)*, how to assist an asthmatic person during an asthma attack *(page 69)* and how to deal with a respiratory allergy *(page 70)*. For techniques on handling a life-threatening respiratory emergency such as choking or arrested breathing, consult the Emergency Guide *(page 8)*. For basic techniques on caring for a family member who is ill or recuperating from an illness, consult the Equipment & Techniques chapter *(page 110)*.

The list of health tips at right covers basic guidelines in helping to prevent respiratory ailments and keep the respiratory system in good condition. Smoking, for example, can be virtually the sole cause of many chronic and deadly respiratory problems. If you are a smoker, stop smoking *(page 70)* and give the delicate organs of your respiratory system a chance at dealing effectively with the myriad infectious agents and airborne pollutants from which it protects your body.

If you must cope with a respiratory ailment in the home, do not hesitate to call for help; medical professionals can answer questions concerning symptoms and treatments. Post the telephone numbers for your physician, local hospital emergency room, ambulance and pharmacy near the telephone; in most regions, dial 911 in the event of a life-threatening emergency. Keep handy the telephone number of an ear, nose and throat specialist recommended by your physician. For general information on respiratory ailments, contact a local chapter of the American Lung Association.

HEALTH TIPS

1. To maintain your overall health and help you prevent an infection of your respiratory system, eat and sleep properly, and avoid stress and excessive use of alcohol.

2. To maintain a healthy respiratory system, do not smoke. If you smoke, make every effort to stop *(page 70)*; if necessary, consult a physician about ways to overcome your habit.

3. To strengthen the respiratory system, get plenty of exercise and fresh air—without overdoing it. Walk rather than drive, for example; or, take up a pastime such as gardening, choosing an activity to suit your tastes and physical strength.

4. To prevent respiratory problems, wear respiratory protection *(page 70)* to do dusty work in the house or to use chemicals that emit hazardous vapors.

5. To prevent respiratory problems, minimize daily exposure to dust and airborne irritants. Vacuum and dust the house, and clean furnace, air conditioner and humidifier filters regularly; if you live in a dusty area, install an air-filtration system.

6. Never suppress a sneeze or cough—they are reflexes that expel dust and bacteria from the respiratory system. Never sneeze with your mouth closed.

7. Breathe through your nose, not your mouth; the nasal cavities are designed to warm and moisten incoming air, and filter out dust and bacteria, minimizing stress on the lungs.

8. In general, consult a physician about any respiratory ailment in an infant, a young child or an elderly person.

9. Consult a physician about a respiratory problem accompanied by a potentially-serious symptom such as: recurrent or persistent cough or sore throat; persistent high fever; swollen neck glands; or, painful, difficult breathing.

10. Minimize the spread of a contagious respiratory infection such as a common cold by: using facial tissues instead of handkerchiefs; covering your nose and mouth to sneeze or cough; washing your hands after contact with an infected person, and washing dishes and linens used by the person.

11. Unless recommended by your physician, avoid using a nonprescription medication to treat a common cold; the medication may have negative side effects.

12. Follow the physician's directions to use any prescription medication; use the amount specified at the prescribed times and report any side effect to the physician.

13. If you suffer from a respiratory ailment such as asthma and use a prescription medication, carry a Medic Alert card or wear a Medic Alert bracelet that will allow a medical professional to identify your condition in an emergency.

14. If you suffer from a major respiratory ailment, consult a physician before undertaking a rigorous physical activity; if recommended, consult a physiotherapist about an exercise program to gradually increase your respiratory capacity.

64

RESPIRATORY SYSTEM

RESPIRATORY SYSTEM

Sinus
Air-filled cavity in bone of forehead and cheek that opens into nasal cavity and mouth. May become blocked and ache due to common cold or respiratory allergy; infection may result in sinusitis requiring medical attention.

Nasal cavity
Air inhaled through nose passes through nasal cavity; cavity wall lined with mucous membrane and tiny hairs (cilia) that warm and moisten air, and trap dust and bacteria before air passes to pharynx. Cavity becomes stuffy and runny due to common cold or respiratory allergy; sneezing is reflex to remove irritants from cavity.

Larynx
Commonly called voice box or Adam's apple. Carries air between pharynx and trachea and houses vocal cords. In adult, infection, smoking or stress may cause inflammation called laryngitis, resulting in hoarseness or loss of voice; in children, infection may cause croup, resulting in hoarse, barking cough.

Pharynx
Commonly called throat. Carries air between nasal cavity or mouth and larynx. Sore throat usually a symptom of infection such as common cold, but may be due to other infections requiring medical attention, especially in children.

Bronchus
Carries air between trachea and bronchioles of a lung. Infection, smoking or pollution may cause inflammation called bronchitis, resulting in wheezy breathing, chronic cough and mucus.

Trachea
Commonly called windpipe. Carries air between larynx and left and right bronchus.

Bronchioles
Branch-like network of passages carry air between bronchus and alveoli—tiny sponge-like air sacs—of lung; alveoli take oxygen out of air and pass it into blood, and take carbon dioxide out of blood and pass it back into air.

Lung
Spongy, sac-like organ comprised of bronchioles and alveoli surrounded by moist membrane called pleura. Expands to fill with oxygen-laden air during inhalation; contracts to push out carbon dioxide-laden air during exhalation. Infection and inflammation of lung parts typically characterized by painful, difficult breathing; usually due to ailment such as asthma, pneumonia or pleurisy.

Diaphragm
Muscle below lungs separates chest from abdomen. Pushed down toward abdomen as lungs expand during inhalation, then pushes up against lungs to help them contract during exhalation. Spasm in diaphragm results in hiccups.

65

Cross-references
Direct you to important information elsewhere in the book.

Health Tips
Cover guidelines for keeping the body system healthy and preventing medical problems.

At the beginning of each chapter, an anatomy diagram of the system that is its focus is presented. Refer to the anatomy diagram to locate and identify the elements of the system, as well as common problems that can be associated with it. The health tips at the start of each chapter cover basic guidelines for preventing family medical problems and practicing healthy living habits at home. Illustrated procedures and information sidebars throughout the chapter feature greater details; for example: preventing respiratory problems by wearing respiratory protection *(page 70)* and cleaning humidifiers *(page 71)*.

Refer to the chapter entitled Equipment & Techniques *(page 110)* for basic techniques on caring at home for a family member who is ill or recuperating from an illness. Read the tips on setting up a recovery room to make a patient as comfortable as possible *(page 112)*. Know how to take the temperature *(page 114)* and monitor the pulse *(page 115)* of a patient. If you ever have questions about a medical problem or doubt your ability to handle it at home, do not hesitate to consult a medical professional. Keep the telephone number of your physician posted near the telephone; in most regions, dial 911 in a medical emergency.

Troubleshooting Guide
To use this chart, locate the entry in column 1 that most closely resembles your problem, then follow the recommended procedures in column 2. Some instructions may be explained in the chart; in other cases, you will be directed to an illustrated procedure sequence or information sidebar.

Medical emergency
Any problem that may be a sign of a medical emergency is indicated in the Troubleshooting Guide.

Name of procedure
You will be referred by the Troubleshooting Guide to the first page of a specific procedure or sidebar.

RESPIRATORY SYSTEM

TROUBLESHOOTING GUIDE

PROBLEM	PROCEDURE
Common cold suspected	Monitor and relieve common cold symptoms (p. 66); consult a physician if no improvement in common cold symptoms within 1 week
Laryngitis suspected: hoarse, squeaky or lost voice	Rest, drink plenty of fluids, stop any smoking (p. 70) and avoid using voice
	Consult a physician if hoarse, squeaky or lost voice lasts more than 4 days
Cough with mucus	Monitor and relieve cough (p. 68)
	Consult a physician if mucus bloody, brown or frothy, or cough lasts more than 1 week
Dry cough	Stop any smoking (p. 70)
	Consult a physician if cough lasts more than 1 week
Sore throat	Monitor and relieve sore throat (p. 68)
	Consult a physician if sore throat lasts more than 2 days
Asthma attack suspected: severe, sudden onset of wheezy breathing	Treat asthma attack (p. 69); seek emergency help ✚ if it lasts more than 30 minutes
	Consult a physician to identify and treat possible allergy (p. 71) or infection
Allergic reaction suspected: sneezing; runny, stuffy nose; itchy, watery, swollen eyes; itchy skin rash; wheezy breathing	For severe, wheezy breathing, treat asthma attack (p. 69); seek emergency help ✚ if it lasts more than 30 minutes
	Consult a physician to identify and treat allergy (p. 71)
Breathing difficult: wheezing	If severe, treat asthma attack (p. 69); seek emergency help ✚ if it lasts more than 30 minutes
	Consult a physician to identify and treat possible allergy (p. 71) or infection
Breathing difficult: pain; breathlessness	If severe, seek emergency help ✚; if necessary, use emergency first aid (p. 8)
	Consult a physician to identify and treat infection
Nosebleed	Stop nosebleed (p. 69)
	Consult a physician if nosebleeds frequent

✚ Medical emergency

TREATING A COMMON COLD

Monitoring and relieving cold symptoms. The common cold is caused by any one of many different viruses that affect the upper respiratory tract—the nose, sinuses and throat. Because you can contract a cold virus through direct contact with a person who has a cold or by inhaling an airborne virus, your risk of contracting a virus is higher if you are regularly exposed to crowded living and working conditions. Whether you develop a cold after contracting a virus depends on whether you are immune to the particular cold virus to which you have been exposed, as well as on your physical condition; if you are stressed, overtired, eat poorly, smoke or have a chronic illness, your chance of developing a cold is greater. Common cold symptoms include: sneezing; stuffy, runny nose; aching, stuffy head; sore throat; cough; fatigue; loss of appetite; and low-grade fever. Once you develop a common cold, there is no "cure" for it—no medication will eliminate the virus or shorten the duration of the cold. In general, take steps to prevent spreading the virus: Avoid direct contact with other people and wash your hands frequently, especially after blowing your nose; avoid handling food that others will eat. Follow the guidelines below to monitor the progress of a common cold and treat its symptoms:

• Get plenty of rest.

• Drink plenty of fluids, especially water and fruit juices; cut back on the intake of milk products which can thicken secretions of mucus and increase congestion.

• If you smoke, reduce stress on the respiratory system by stopping smoking (page 70).

• Check the neck glands (page 56) and consult a physician if the neck glands are swollen.

• Monitor temperature (page 114) and consult a physician if a fever persists for more than a few days, rises above 101° Fahrenheit or is accompanied by chills.

• Relieve aches and reduce fever by using a nonprescription pain-reliever (page 121) and consult a physician if there is persistent or severe pain in the teeth, sinuses or ear.

• Relieve congestion by using a humidifier and saline nose drops; for an infant, also a nasal aspirator (page 67).

• Monitor and relieve any sore throat (page 68).

• Monitor and relieve any cough (page 69) and consult a physician if coughing is uncontrolled or excessive, or is accompanied by difficult, painful breathing.

• Consult a physician if there is no improvement in symptoms after 7 days or if any symptom remains after 14 days.

66

RESPIRATORY SYSTEM

RELIEVING CONGESTION

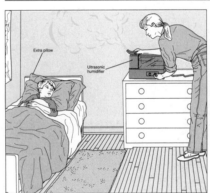

Extra pillow

Ultrasonic humidifier

Using a humidifier. To help relieve the congestion of a common cold, use a humidifier such as the ultrasonic type shown; extra humidity can help loosen mucus secretions and clear blocked sinuses, stuffy nasal passages and congested breathing. Use the humidifier wherever a person with a cold rests or sleeps, ensuring you clean it daily (page 71). Following the manufacturer's instructions, set up the humidifier on a steady surface near the person, adjusting any nozzle on it (left) to direct a steady flow of mist into the air around the person. **Caution:** Never position a humidifier where a child can grab or tip it. To provide additional relief from congestion during rest or sleep, use an extra pillow to elevate the head slightly.

To provide spot-relief from blocked sinuses and stuffy nasal passages, use a hot compress. Soak a clean facecloth in hot—not scalding—water and wring it out, then fold it into a pad and wrap it with a towel. Hold the compress gently against one side of the nose to cover the cheek and eye, leaving it in place for 10 minutes. Reheat the compress and do the same on the other side of the nose.

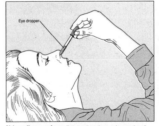

Eye dropper

Using saline nose drops. To help relieve the nasal congestion of a common cold, use a fresh solution of saline nose drops in each nostril twice a day. Fill a clean eye dropper with a cool saline solution of 1 teaspoon of salt per cup of boiling water. Tilting the head back as far as possible, insert the tip of the eye dropper into a nostril (above) and squeeze 3 drops of the solution into it. Without tilting the head forward, do the same for the other nostril. Keep the head tilted back for 2 to 3 minutes before tilting it forward again. Alternatively, buy nonprescription saline nose drops at a pharmacy and follow the manufacturer's instructions to use them.

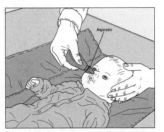

Aspirator

Using a nasal aspirator. To relieve nasal congestion in an infant, lay him on his back; if necessary, have a helper hold the infant's hands to prevent fidgeting. Administer saline nose drops (step left), then clear each nostril twice using a nasal aspirator. To use the aspirator, squeeze its bulb, then gently insert its nozzle into the tip of a nostril (above). **Caution:** Never insert the nozzle without first squeezing the bulb. To extract mucus from the nostril, slowly release the bulb. To drain the aspirator, squeeze the bulb to expel the mucus into a facial tissue, then use a fresh tissue to wipe the nozzle clean. After using the aspirator, wash and rinse it well.

67

Information sidebars
Provide detailed information on handling and preventing problems with the body system.

Lead-ins
Bold lead-ins summarize each procedure or highlight the key action shown in the illustration.

EMERGENCY GUIDE

Preventing family medical problems. No family is ever immune to medical problems. Fortunately, many household medical emergencies are not life-threatening; with basic first-aid techniques, you can be prepared to handle most of them. However, in the event of a life-threatening medical emergency, the correct action taken quickly can maintain a life until emergency help arrives. Identify potential medical emergencies among your family members and find out where to obtain emergency medical help *(page 9)*. Familiarize yourself with the signs and symptoms of life-threatening medical emergencies included in this chapter; practice monitoring the vital life signs of breathing and pulse *(page 12)* before an emergency occurs.

The Troubleshooting Guide on pages 10 and 11 places procedures for life-threatening family medical emergencies at your fingertips; it provides you with quick-action steps to take and refers you to pages 12 to 29 for more detailed information. Study the steps to take on handling an unconscious adult or child *(page 12)* and an unconscious infant up to 12 months old *(page 19)*. Familiarize yourself with the procedures for administering artificial respiration to an adult or child *(page 14)* and an infant *(page 20)*. Know how to treat a choking adult or child *(page 16)* and a choking infant *(page 21)*. Learn the procedure for controlling bleeding *(page 13)*. Study the signs of shock that may accompany a medical emergency and how to handle the victim of it *(page 23)*. Practice placing a person in the recovery position *(page 22)* as well as moving a conscious person *(page 29)*.

The list of safety tips at right covers basic guidelines to help you keep family medical emergencies from occurring; refer to page 28 for information on preventing accidental poisoning. To be fully prepared for a life-threatening medical emergency, you should take a course in cardiopulmonary resuscitation (CPR), offered by the American Red Cross and the American Heart Association. CPR requires hands-on training and the expert guidance of professional instructors; administer it only if you are qualified. Keep a well-stocked first-aid kit on hand in your home *(page 110)* and know how to use the supplies it contains.

When confronted with a life-threatening medical emergency, stay calm; the first step in providing assistance to a victim is clear thinking and an unpanicked response. First treat the victim, then telephone for emergency medical help; if possible, instruct someone to make the call for you. Do not move a victim if you suspect that he has sustained a spinal injury *(page 23)*. If you must rescue a victim from contact with a live electrical current, do not touch him or the electrical source; use a wooden broom handle or other wooden implement to knock him free, then monitor his vital life signs *(page 27)*. Do not attempt to remove an embedded object from the skin; immobilize it and control bleeding from the wound *(page 13)*. In the event of any medical emergency, do not hesitate to call for medical assistance; even in situations that may not be life-threatening, medical professionals can answer your questions about proper emergency techniques and follow-up treatment.

SAFETY TIPS

1. Prepare yourself and your family members to handle a medical emergency by posting emergency telephone numbers at each telephone of your household *(page 9)*.

2. Prepare others to handle a medical emergency involving you or a family member with medical identification *(page 9)*.

3. Equip yourself to handle a medical emergency by taking courses in first aid and cardiopulmonary resuscitation (CPR); for information, contact your local branch of the American Red Cross or American Heart Association.

4. Do not attempt to move a victim if you suspect a spinal injury *(page 23)* or he complains of extreme pain; cover him with a blanket to keep him warm and immediately call for emergency help.

5. If a victim has no pulse or his pulse is weak or irregular, administer CPR only if you are qualified. An unqualified person attempting to administer CPR risks harming the victim; place him in the recovery position *(page 22)* and immediately call for emergency help.

6. Take measures to prevent an ingested poisoning *(page 28)* and keep a bottle of syrup of ipecac on hand; administer it to a victim of ingested poisoning to induce vomiting only if instructed by a medical professional.

7. Childproof your home. Store all medication and harmful household products well out of the reach of children—behind a locked door or in a locked drawer. Ensure that any swimming pool is fenced in and that the gate is kept locked when the area is unsupervised. Take the door off a refrigerator or freezer when storing or discarding it in order to prevent a child from trapping himself and possibly suffocating.

8. To help prevent injuries from accidental falls, keep all stairways well-lighted and free of clutter. Clear snow and ice off walkways. Install handrails and no-slip rubber mats in bathtubs and shower stalls. Work safely when using a ladder; set it up properly and do not overreach.

9. Put tools and equipment safely away as soon as you have finished your work; do not leave them out where they can be stumbled over or reached by children.

10. Do not use any electrical unit near a toilet, bathtub, shower or sink, or around any source of water. Never operate an electrical unit in wet or damp conditions.

11. During a heat wave or unusually high temperatures, avoid strenuous physical activity. If you go outdoors, stay in the shade; wear a hat and light-colored clothing.

12. During extreme low temperatures, stay indoors. If you must venture outdoors, dress for the weather to guard against hypothermia and frostbite of exposed skin or extremities—your nose, ears, face, hands and feet.

13. Keep a well-stocked first-aid kit *(page 110)* on hand in a convenient, accessible place in your home.

IDENTIFYING MEDICAL EMERGENCIES

Wearing medical identification. Quick action in the event of a medical emergency can save a life—only if it is the correct action, based on the right information. To help ensure that the correct action can be taken quickly in a medical emergency, you and your family members should wear a medical identification bracelet *(right, top)* or pendant and carry a medical identification card for any diagnosed medical condition, known allergy or sensitivity, or needed prescribed medication.

Typical medical conditions, allergies and sensitivities, and prescribed medications for which medical identification should be worn and carried are listed in the chart *(right, bottom)*; identification is also available and recommended for wearers of contact lenses. The Medic-Alert Foundation provides medical identification, making available urgent information on a registered individual to emergency personnel through its network. For information on obtaining medical identification, consult your physician or a pharmacist, or call 1-800-ID-ALERT.

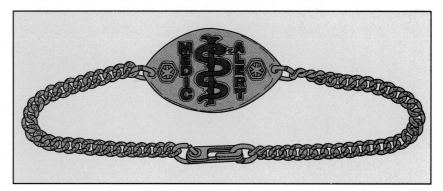

MEDICAL CONDITION	ALLERGY/SENSITIVITY	PRESCRIBED MEDICATION
• Alzheimer's disease	• Aspirin	• Anti-anginal
• Angina	• Codeine	• Anticoagulant
• Bleeding disorder	• Horse serum	• Anticonvulsant
• Diabetes/insulin dependent	• Lidocaine	• Antihistamine, prolonged use
• Diabetes/non-insulin dependent	• Novocaine	• Beta blocker
• Seizure disorder	• Penicillin	• Cortisone or steroids
• Hypertension	• Tetracycline	
	• Insect stings	
	• X-ray dyes	
	• Iodine	

GETTING HELP IN MEDICAL EMERGENCIES

Calling for medical help. Precious seconds can be saved in a medical emergency if you know where to call for assistance—and make the difference in a life-threatening situation. With the proper information on obtaining help, you can prepare yourself and your family members to handle an emergency.

• **911.** In most regions, you should dial 911 in the event of any life-threatening emergency; be prepared to calmly provide information on the nature of the emergency and your specific location. If necessary, dial 911 and leave the telephone handset off the hook, keeping the line open for it to be traced; teach a young child to follow this procedure in an emergency.

• **Emergency medical service (EMS).** For a life-threatening medical emergency such as a heart attack, you can telephone a private company for ambulance service or your local community EMS unit. By calling EMS, care can be provided by a qualified team of emergency technicians or paramedics, supervised by a physician of the emergency department at a local hospital; transportation to the hospital is also supplied.

• **Fire and police departments.** If you live in a community without an established EMS unit or in a large urban center, you can telephone your local fire or police department for any life-threatening emergency. Many fire and police departments have rescue units of personnel trained in life-support techniques and other emergency medical procedures; most can provide speedy transportation to the emergency department of the nearest hospital.

Research the emergency medical resources of your local community, finding out the services that are available and how they can be obtained. Post a list of telephone numbers to use in a medical emergency at a convenient, accessible spot near each telephone of your household; include the following:

• **Hospital emergency department.** For a medical emergency that is not immediately life-threatening, you can go directly to the emergency department of your local hospital. A hospital emergency department provides medical services 24 hours a day and is usually staffed at any time by at least one physician. If possible, call ahead before leaving for the hospital, prepared to provide information on the nature of the emergency and likely time of your arrival.

• **Physician and dentist.** Having your own physician and dentist ensures that your medical and dental history is on record in one place—for referral in emergency and non-emergency situations. Your own physician and dentist can usually arrange an appointment on short notice in an emergency; they can also supply answers to your questions on the telephone.

• **Poison control center.** If you suspect a poisoning, telephone your local poison control center for emergency instructions; be prepared to calmly provide information on the victim's age and weight as well as the type and amount of poison taken. Your local poison control center can also provide up-to-date information on poison prevention and the safe disposal of poisonous substances.

TROUBLESHOOTING GUIDE

PROBLEM	PROCEDURE
Loss of consciousness suspected: loss of muscle, eye or speech control	Check victim's responsiveness: adult or child (p. 12); infant (p. 19)
	If victim does not respond, immediately have someone call for emergency help
	Monitor victim's vital life signs: adult or child (p. 12); infant (p. 19)
	If no pulse or pulse weak or irregular, administer cardiopulmonary resuscitation only if qualified
	If no breathing or breathing shallow or uneven, administer artifical respiration: adult or child (p. 14); infant (p. 20)
	Place victim in recovery position (p. 22)
Profuse bleeding; spurting, bright red blood or gushing, burgundy blood	Immediately have someone call for emergency help
	Control bleeding (p. 13)
	Check victim's responsiveness and monitor vital life signs: adult or child (p. 12); infant (p. 19)
	Place victim in recovery position (p. 22); if necessary, transport conscious victim (p. 29)
Choking: gagging, blue in face	Immediately have someone call for emergency help
	Treat choking victim: adult or child (p. 16); self-help (p. 17); infant (p. 21)
	Check victim's responsiveness and monitor vital life signs; adult or child (p. 12); infant (p. 19)
	If no pulse or pulse weak or irregular, administer cardiopulmonary resuscitation only if qualified
	If no breathing or breathing shallow or uneven, administer artifical respiration (p. 14)
	Place victim in recovery position (p. 22); if necessary, transport conscious victim (p. 29)
Spinal injury suspected: fall from roof, ladder or top of stairs; blow to head, neck or back	Do not move victim; immediately have someone call for emergency help
	Treat victim of spinal injury (p. 23)
	Check victim's responsiveness and monitor vital life signs (p. 12)
Shock suspected: trauma; injury; illness; sudden emotional upset	Immediately have someone call for emergency help
	Treat victim of shock (p. 23)
	Check victim's responsiveness and monitor vital life signs (p. 12)
	If no pulse or pulse weak or irregular, administer cardiopulmonary resuscitation only if qualified
	If no breathing or breathing shallow or uneven, administer artifical respiration (p. 14)
	Place victim in recovery position (p. 22); if necessary, transport conscious victim (p. 29)
Heart attack suspected: tightness or pain across chest; labored breathing; weak or irregular pulse; cold or clammy skin	Immediately have someone call for emergency help
	Treat victim of heart attack (p. 24)
	Check victim's responsiveness and monitor vital life signs (p. 12)
	If no pulse or pulse weak or irregular, administer cardiopulmonary resuscitation only if qualified
	If no breathing or breathing shallow or uneven, administer artifical respiration (p. 14)
	Place victim in recovery position (p. 22); if necessary, transport conscious victim (p. 29)
Stroke suspected: disorientation; paralysis or weakness on one side of body; speaking, swallowing or breathing difficulty	Immediately have someone call for emergency help
	Treat victim of stroke (p. 24)
	Check victim's responsiveness and monitor vital life signs (p. 12)
	If no pulse or pulse weak or irregular, administer cardiopulmonary resuscitation only if qualified
	If no breathing or breathing shallow or uneven, administer artifical respiration (p. 14)
	Place victim in recovery position (p. 22); if necessary, transport conscious victim (p. 29)
Allergic reaction suspected: extreme body response to contact with allergen	Immediately have someone call for emergency help
	Treat victim of allergic reaction (p. 25)
	Check victim's responsiveness and monitor vital life signs: adult or child (p. 12); infant (p. 19)
	If no pulse or pulse weak or irregular, administer cardiopulmonary resuscitation only if qualified
	If no breathing or breathing shallow or uneven, administer artifical respiration: adult or child (p. 14); infant (p. 20)
	Place victim in recovery position (p. 22); if necessary, transport conscious victim (p. 29)

PROBLEM	PROCEDURE
Diabetic emergency suspected: insulin shock due to insufficient sugar; diabetic coma due to excess sugar (insufficient insulin)	Immediately have someone call for emergency help
	Treat victim of diabetic emergency (p. 25)
	Check victim's responsiveness and monitor vital life signs: adult or child (p. 12); infant (p. 19)
	If no pulse or pulse weak or irregular, administer cardiopulmonary resuscitation only if qualified
	If no breathing or breathing shallow or uneven, administer artifical respiration: adult or child (p. 14); infant (p. 20)
	Place victim in recovery position (p. 22); if necessary, transport conscious victim (p. 29)
Hypothermia or frostbite suspected: prolonged exposure to extreme cold	Treat victim of exposure to extreme cold (p. 26); if necessary, transport conscious victim (p. 29)
	Check victim's responsiveness: adult or child (p. 12); infant (p. 19)
	If victim does not respond, immediately have someone call for emergency help
	Monitor victim's vital life signs: adult or child (p. 12); infant (p. 19)
	If no pulse or pulse weak or irregular, administer cardiopulmonary resuscitation only if qualified
	If no breathing or breathing shallow or uneven, administer artifical respiration: adult or child (p. 14); infant (p. 20)
	Place victim in recovery position (p. 22)
Heat stroke suspected: prolonged exposure to extreme heat	Treat victim of exposure to extreme heat (p. 26); if necessary, transport conscious victim (p. 29)
	Check victim's responsiveness: adult or child (p. 12); infant (p. 19)
	If victim does not respond, immediately have someone call for emergency help
	Monitor victim's vital life signs: adult or child (p. 12); infant (p. 19)
	If no pulse or pulse weak or irregular, administer cardiopulmonary resuscitation only if qualified
	If no breathing or breathing shallow or uneven, administer artifical respiration: adult or child (p. 14); infant (p. 20)
	Place victim in recovery position (p. 22)
Burn	Treat victim of burn (p. 27)
	Check victim's responsiveness: adult or child (p. 12); infant (p. 19)
	If victim does not respond, immediately have someone call for emergency help
	Monitor victim's vital life signs: adult or child (p. 12); infant (p. 19)
	If no pulse or pulse weak or irregular, administer cardiopulmonary resuscitation only if qualified
	If no breathing or breathing shallow or uneven, administer artifical respiration: adult or child (p. 14); infant (p. 20)
	Place victim in recovery position (p. 22); if necessary, transport conscious victim (p. 29)
Electrical shock	If victim immobilized by live current, knock him free using wooden implement (p. 27)
	Immediately have someone call for emergency help
	Monitor victim's vital life signs: adult or child (p. 12); infant (p. 19) .
	If no pulse or pulse weak or irregular, administer cardiopulmonary resuscitation only if qualified
	If no breathing or breathing shallow or uneven, administer artifical respiration: adult or child (p. 14); infant (p. 20)
	Place victim in recovery position (p. 22); if necessary, transport conscious victim (p. 29)
Poison ingestion	Treat victim of poison ingestion (p. 28)
	Check victim's responsiveness: adult or child (p. 12); infant (p. 19)
	If victim does not respond, immediately have someone call for emergency help
	Monitor victim's vital life signs: adult or child (p. 12); infant (p. 19)
	If no pulse or pulse weak or irregular, administer cardiopulmonary resuscitation only if qualified
	If no breathing or breathing shallow or uneven, administer artifical respiration: adult or child (p. 14); infant (p. 20)
	Place victim in recovery position (p. 22); if necessary, transport conscious victim (p. 29)
	Take steps to prevent ingested poisoning (p. 28)

TREATING AN UNCONSCIOUS VICTIM (ADULT OR CHILD)

Monitoring a victim's vital life signs.
In the event of a major medical emergency, a victim can lose consciousness—a sign of interference with the nervous or circulatory system. A victim may have suffered a loss of consciousness if his eyes do not open or open only to speech or pain, his response to speech is silence or confusion, and his muscles do not respond or respond only to pain. If you suspect that a victim has suffered a loss of consciousness, immediately deal with him, then call for emergency help; if possible, instruct someone to make the call for you. If the victim is an infant, check his responsiveness and monitor his vital life signs (page 19). Otherwise, reassure the victim that medical help is on the way and check his responsiveness (step 1). While waiting for emergency help to arrive, keep others from crowding around the victim and monitor his vital life signs—the ABCs of emergency care:

- A for airway—check that there is an open airway (step 2)

- B for breathing—check that there is breathing (step 3)

- C for circulation—check that there is a pulse (step 4) and control any bleeding (page 13).

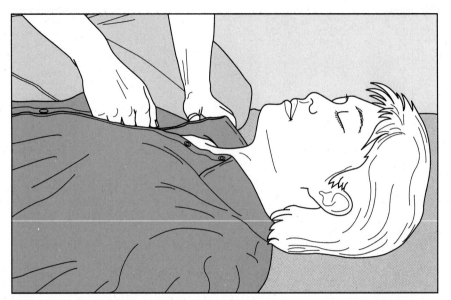

1 **Checking for responsiveness. Caution:** If you suspect that the victim has suffered a spinal injury (page 23), do not move him. Otherwise, roll the victim onto his back and loosen his clothing at the neck, chest and waist. To check the responsiveness of the victim, kneel beside him and ask if help is needed. If the victim does not respond, lightly slap his cheeks, then pinch an earlobe and ask again if help is needed. If the victim again does not respond, gently roll the knuckles of one hand against his breastbone (above). If the victim still does not respond, assume that he has suffered a loss of consciousness and immediately have someone call for emergency help, then check that the victim's airway is open (step 2).

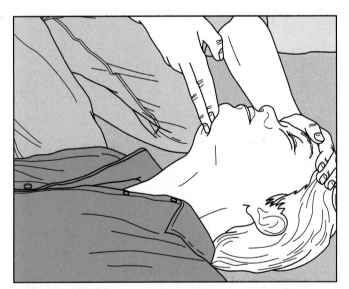

2 **Checking for an open airway.** In many instances, the victim can breathe on his own if his airway is open. **Caution:** If you suspect that the victim has suffered a spinal injury (page 23), wait for emergency help to arrive and do not move him. Otherwise, open the victim's airway by placing the index and middle fingers of one hand under his chin and lifting it, then gently push down on his forehead with the other hand (above); this action raises his lower jaw and draws his tongue away from the back of his throat. Drop the victim's lower jaw, opening his mouth, then check for breathing (step 3).

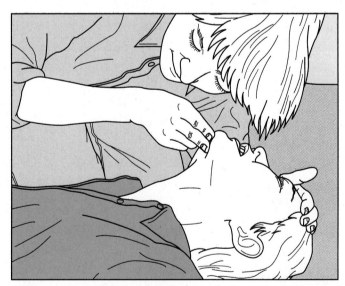

3 **Checking for breathing.** To check for breathing, lower your head, placing your ear and cheek within 1/2 inch of the victim's mouth to hear and feel air being exhaled (above). Look closely for a rise and fall of the victim's chest as he inhales and exhales—indicating he is breathing. Maintain this position for 5 to 10 seconds, looking, listening and feeling for signs of breathing. Normal breathing at rest is quiet and regular with an even rhythm. If there is no breathing or the breathing is shallow or uneven, immediately administer artifical respiration (page 14). Otherwise, check for a pulse (step 4).

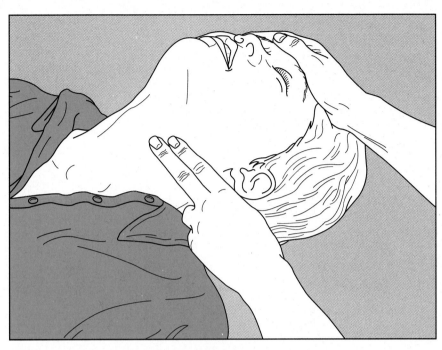

4 Checking for a pulse. Keeping the victim's airway open, take his pulse at the carotid artery of his neck on the side closest to you; do not reach across his windpipe. To locate the artery, place the tips of the index and middle fingers of one hand on the side of the victim's windpipe, about halfway between his chin and collarbone. Press gently into the space between the victim's windpipe and the neck muscle *(left)* to feel for the pulse, maintaining this position for 5 to 10 seconds. A normal pulse is strong and regular. If there is no pulse or the pulse is weak or irregular, immediately administer cardiopulmonary resuscitation (CPR) only if you are qualified. Otherwise, control any bleeding *(step below)* and wait for emergency help to arrive.

CONTROLLING BLEEDING

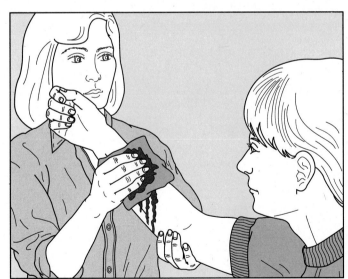

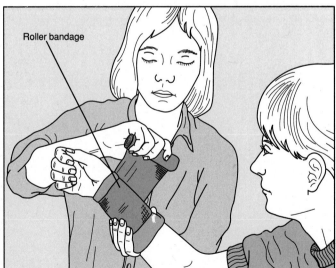

Roller bandage

Applying direct pressure to stop bleeding. Profuse, rapid bleeding can occur if a major artery or vein *(page 56)* is severed. If the bleeding is profuse or rapid, immediately have someone call for emergency help, then monitor the victim's vital life signs *(page 12)*. To help stop the bleeding, apply direct pressure to the wound with a gauze dressing or a clean cloth and, if possible, elevate the injury *(above, left)*. **Caution:** If you suspect that the victim has suffered a spinal injury *(page 23)*, wait for emergency help to arrive and do not

move him. Direct pressure applied to the wound should help to stop the flow of blood and allow it to clot. If the dressing or cloth becomes blood-soaked, add another one over the first one; avoid lifting the dressing or cloth to inspect the wound. If necessary, also wrap the wound with a roller bandage *(above, right)* for added direct pressure. Continue applying direct pressure and elevating the injury until the bleeding stops. If the bleeding persists or the wound is deep or gaping, call for emergency help and monitor the victim's vital life signs.

ADMINISTERING ARTIFICAL RESPIRATION (ADULT OR CHILD)

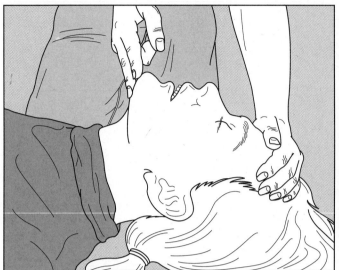

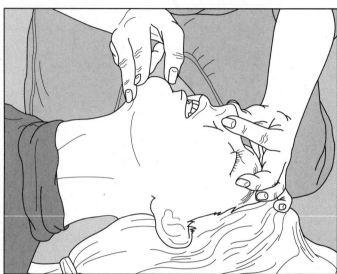

1 **Opening the airway.** Immediately have someone call for emergency help, then monitor the victim's vital life signs *(page 12)*. **Caution:** If you suspect that the victim has suffered a spinal injury *(page 23)*, wait for emergency help to arrive and do not move him. Otherwise, carefully place the victim on his back and loosen his clothing at the neck, chest and waist. If the victim is not breathing or his breathing is shallow or uneven, open his airway. Place the index and middle fingers of one hand under the victim's chin and lift it, then gently push down on his forehead

with the other hand *(above, left)*. Drop the victim's lower jaw, opening his mouth. If you can see that there is an obstruction in the victim's mouth, carefully remove it *(step 6)*. Otherwise, check for breathing *(page 12)*. If there is still no breathing or the breathing is shallow or uneven, hold the victim's lower jaw to keep his mouth open and pinch his nostrils to close them *(above, right)*, then blow air into his lungs *(step 2)*. Otherwise, place the victim in the recovery position *(page 22)*.

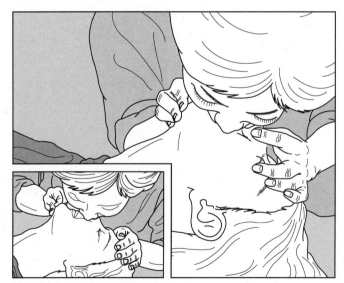

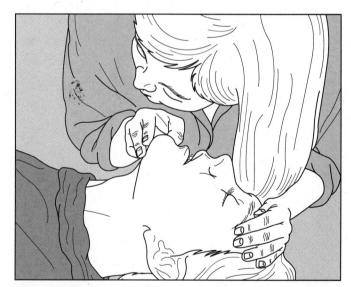

2 **Blowing air into the lungs.** Still holding the victim's lower jaw to keep his mouth open and pinching his nostrils to close them, take a deep breath and press your open mouth over his mouth, forming a tight seal *(above)*. Deliver the full breath slowly, breathing into the victim only enough air to make his chest rise. Remove your mouth to take another deep breath and deliver it the same way. If the victim has a mouth injury or you cannot form a tight seal over his mouth, raise his lower jaw to close his mouth and deliver two full breaths slowly through his nostrils *(inset)*. If the victim vomits, prevent him from choking *(step 4)*; otherwise, check for breathing *(step 3)*.

3 **Checking for breathing.** Break contact with the victim to let air flow into his lungs, then take a deep breath and check for breathing *(page 12)*, dropping his lower jaw to open his mouth *(above)*. If there is no breathing or the breathing is shallow or uneven, blow air into the victim's lungs again *(step 2)*. If there is still no breathing, deliver abdominal thrusts *(step 5)*. Otherwise, continue to blow air into the victim's lungs, delivering one full breath slowly every 5 seconds; for a child, every 4 seconds. When the victim can breathe on his own, place him in the recovery position *(page 22)*. Monitor the victim's vital life signs *(page 12)* until emergency help arrives.

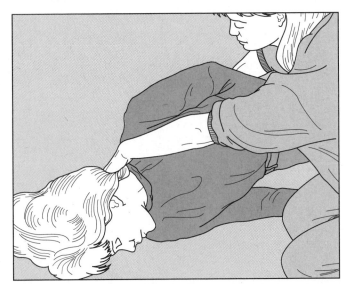

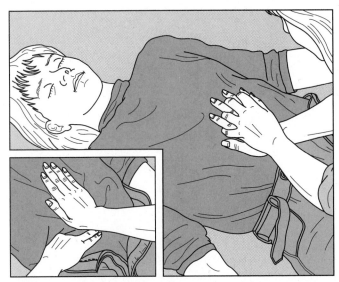

4 **Preventing choking.** During the administering of artifical respiration, air may enter the stomach of the victim and cause him to vomit. **Caution:** Do not attempt to expel air from the victim's stomach by pressing down on it. To prevent the victim from choking, firmly support his head and neck, then gently roll him onto his side *(above)*. Open the victim's mouth with the index finger and thumb of one hand, then sweep the inside of his mouth to clear it using the index finger of the other hand. Supporting the victim's head and neck, carefully roll him onto his back to open his airway *(step 1)* and blow air into his lungs *(step 2)*.

5 **Delivering abdominal thrusts.** An obstruction can lodge in the airway of the victim, interfering with his ability to breathe. To dislodge an obstruction, straddle the victim's thighs and deliver abdominal thrusts. Place the heel of one hand on the victim's abdomen, above his navel by about the width of two fingers and well below the tip of his breastbone *(inset)*. Without moving the heel of your hand, interlace the fingers with the fingers of your other hand. Press firmly with the heel of your hand, rolling inward and upward in one short, quick thrust *(above)*; do not apply pressure with your fingers. Deliver four thrusts, then check for the obstruction *(step 6)*.

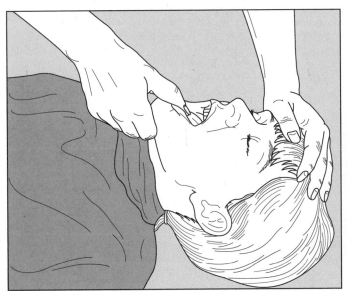

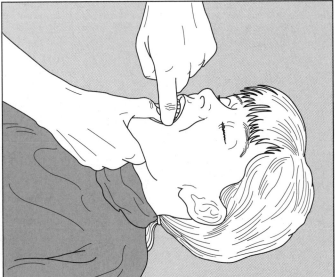

6 **Checking for an obstruction.** To check the victim's mouth for an obstruction, open it with the index finger and thumb of one hand, then sweep the inside of it to clear it using a finger of the other hand. Crossing your finger over your thumb, place your thumb against the victim's lower teeth and your finger against his upper teeth; uncross your finger and your thumb, opening his mouth. Hold the victim's lower jaw and press his tongue down with your thumb to keep his mouth open *(above, left)*.

Carefully pull the obstruction out of the victim's mouth, running your index finger in along one cheek, across the throat and back out along the other cheek *(above, right)*; for a small child, use your baby finger. Sweep the victim's mouth carefully to avoid pushing the obstruction farther into it or down his throat. When the obstruction is removed from the victim's mouth, check for breathing *(step 3)*. Otherwise, continue delivering abdominal thrusts *(step 5)* and checking for an obstruction until emergency help arrives.

TREATING A CHOKING VICTIM (ADULT OR CHILD)

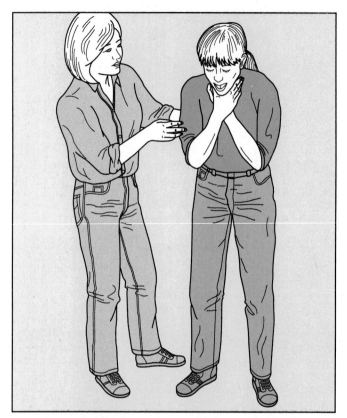

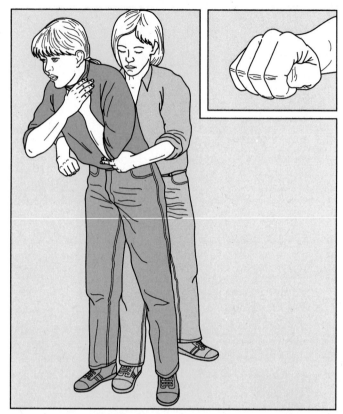

1 Preparing to assist the victim. A choking victim usually puts his hands to his throat; this is recognized as the distress sign for choking. A choking victim may have an obstruction lodged in his windpipe, interfering with his ability to breathe. Immediately have someone call for emergency help. If you are the victim, dislodge the obstruction with self-help *(page 17)*. Otherwise, encourage the victim to dislodge the obstruction by coughing *(above)*. If the victim cannot cough or coughs only weakly and cannot speak, brace him *(step 2)*.

2 Bracing the victim. If the victim loses consciousness, act quickly to clear the obstruction *(step 4)*. Otherwise, brace the victim by standing behind him with one leg between his legs, then wrap your arms under his arms and around his waist *(above)*. If the victim is pregnant or obese or you otherwise cannot reach around his waist, provide assistance by bracing him and administering chest thrusts *(page 18)*. To prepare to deliver abdominal thrusts to the victim, make a fist with one hand, keeping your thumb tucked inside your fingers *(inset)*.

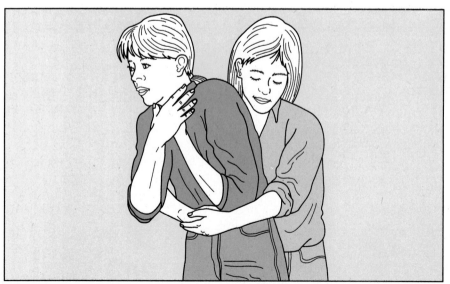

3 Delivering abdominal thrusts. Keeping your thumb tucked inside your fingers, place your fist thumb-first against the victim's abdomen, above his navel by about the width of two fingers and well below his rib cage. Without moving your fist, grasp it firmly with your other hand and press it into the victim's abdomen, rolling inward and upward in one short, quick thrust *(left)*; do not apply pressure with your fingers. Without opening your fist or shifting its position, continue to deliver abdominal thrusts to the victim until the obstruction is removed. If the victim loses consciousness, act quickly to clear the obstruction *(step 4)*. Otherwise, place the victim in the recovery position *(page 22)*.

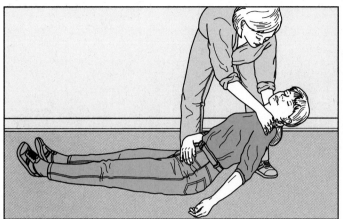
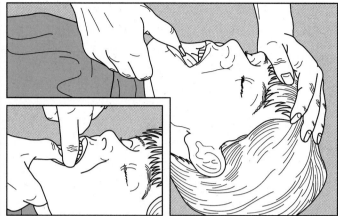

4 **Clearing the obstruction.** If the victim loses consciousness, carefully lower him to the ground, placing him on his back; be sure that you firmly support his head and neck *(above, left)*. Open the victim's mouth with the index finger and thumb of one hand, then sweep the inside of it to clear it using a finger of the other hand. Crossing your finger over your thumb, place your thumb against the victim's lower teeth and your finger against his upper teeth; uncross your finger and your thumb, opening his mouth. Hold the victim's lower jaw and press his tongue

down with your thumb to keep his mouth open *(above, right)*. Carefully pull the obstruction out of the victim's mouth, running your index finger in along one cheek, across the throat and back out along the other cheek *(inset)*; for a small child, use your baby finger. Sweep the victim's mouth carefully to avoid pushing the obstruction farther into it or down his throat. When the obstruction is removed, monitor the victim's vital life signs *(page 12)*. Otherwise, continue to deliver abdominal thrusts and check for the obstruction *(page 15)* until emergency help arrives.

SELF-HELP FOR A CHOKING VICTIM

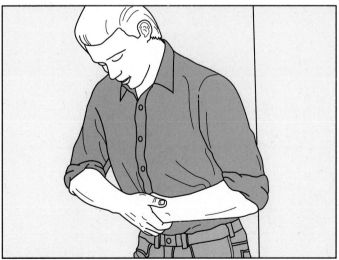
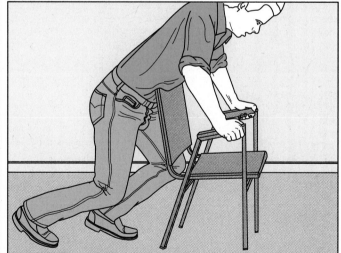

Self-delivering abdominal thrusts. Immediately have someone call for emergency help; if you are alone, dial 911 and leave the handset off the hook. Brace yourself by standing against a wall, then make a fist with your non-dominant hand, keeping your thumb tucked inside your fingers. Place your fist thumb-first against your abdomen, above your navel by about the width of two fingers and well below your rib cage. Without moving your fist, grasp it firmly with your other hand and press it into your abdomen,

rolling inward and upward in one short, quick thrust *(above, left)*; do not press with your fingers. Without opening your fist or shifting its position, continue to deliver abdominal thrusts until the obstruction is removed. Or, assist yourself using the edge of a chair, table, sink, fence or other firm object. Gripping the object firmly with both hands, place your abdomen against its edge and press yourself into it, rolling inward and downward in one short, quick thrust *(above, right)*. Continue the same way until the obstruction is removed.

TREATING A CHOKING VICTIM (OBESE OR PREGNANT ADULT)

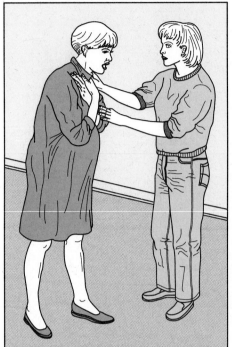 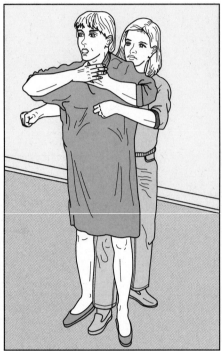 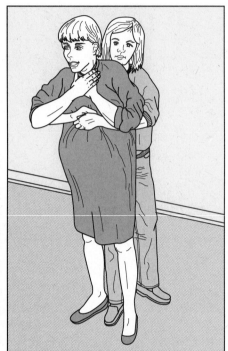

1 Preparing to assist the victim.
A choking victim usually puts his hands to his throat; this is recognized as the distress sign for choking. Immediately have someone call for emergency help. If you are the victim, dislodge the obstruction with self-help *(page 17)*. Otherwise, encourage the victim to dislodge the obstruction by coughing *(above)*. If the victim cannot cough or coughs only weakly and cannot speak, brace him *(step 2)*.

2 Bracing the victim. If the victim loses consciousness, act quickly to clear the obstruction *(step 4)*. Otherwise, brace the victim by standing behind him with one leg between his legs, then wrap your arms under his arms and around his chest *(above)*. Find the midpoint of the victim's breastbone by tracing the curve of the rib cage, then make a fist with one hand, keeping your thumb tucked inside your fingers.

3 Delivering chest thrusts.
Keeping your thumb tucked inside your fingers, place your fist thumb-first against the midpoint of the victim's breastbone, centered on it just below his armpits and above his rib cage. Without moving your fist, grasp it firmly with your other hand and press it straight into the victim's chest cavity in one short, quick thrust *(above)*; do not apply pressure with your fingers.

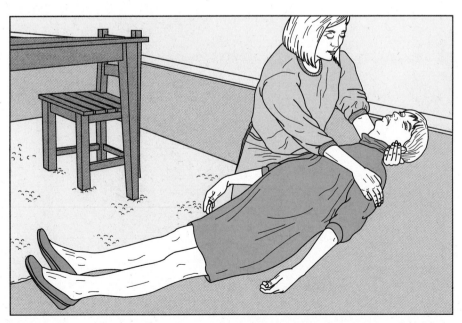

4 Clearing the obstruction.
Without opening your fist or shifting its position, continue to deliver chest thrusts to the victim until the obstruction is removed. Then, place the victim in the recovery position *(page 22)*. If the victim loses consciousness, carefully lower him to the ground, placing him on his back; be sure that you firmly support his head and neck *(left)*. Check for the obstruction and deliver abdominal thrusts *(page 15)*. **Caution:** Do not deliver abdominal thrusts if the victim is pregnant. When the obstruction is removed, monitor the victim's vital life signs *(page 12)* until emergency help arrives.

TREATING AN UNCONSCIOUS VICTIM (INFANT)

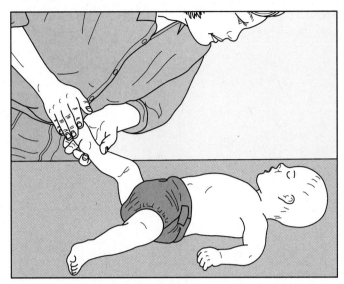

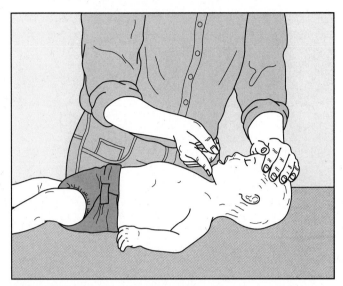

1 **Checking for responsiveness.** Carefully place the infant on his back and loosen any clothing at his neck, chest and waist. To check the responsiveness of the infant, gently shake him. If the infant does not respond, tap his foot *(above)* or hand and shout loudly. If the infant still does not respond, assume that he has suffered a loss of consciousness and immediately have someone call for emergency help, then check that the infant's airway is open *(step 2)*.

2 **Checking for an open airway.** In many instances, the infant can breathe on his own if his airway is open. Tilt the infant's head back, gently lifting his chin with a finger of one hand and pushing down on his forehead with the other hand *(above)*; this action raises his lower jaw and draws his tongue away from the back of his throat. **Caution:** Overextending the infant's neck can cause an injury. Drop the infant's lower jaw, opening his mouth, then check for breathing *(step 3)*.

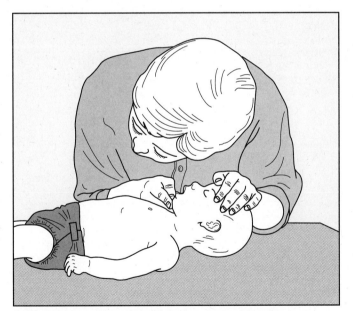

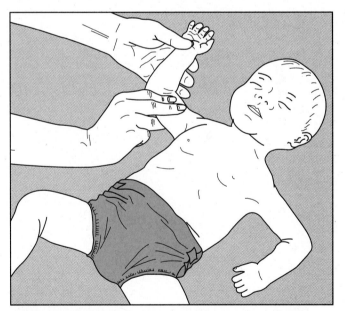

3 **Checking for breathing.** To check for breathing, lower your head, placing your ear and cheek within 1/2 inch of the infant's mouth to hear and feel air being exhaled *(above)*. Look closely for a rise and fall of the infant's chest as he inhales and exhales—indicating he is breathing. Maintain this position for 5 to 10 seconds, looking, listening and feeling for signs of breathing. Normal breathing at rest is quiet and regular with an even rhythm. If there is no breathing or the breathing is shallow or uneven, immediately administer artifical respiration *(page 20)*. Otherwise, check for a pulse *(step 4)*.

4 **Checking for a pulse.** Take the infant's pulse at the brachial artery of his upper arm. Place the tips of the index and middle fingers of one hand on the inside of the infant's upper arm, midway between his shoulder and elbow. Press gently into the infant's upper arm *(above)* to feel for the pulse, maintaining this position for 5 to 10 seconds. A normal pulse is strong and regular. If there is no pulse or the pulse is weak or irregular, immediately administer cardiopulmonary resuscitation (CPR) only if you are qualified. Otherwise, control any bleeding *(page 13)* and wait for emergency help to arrive.

ADMINISTERING ARTIFICIAL RESPIRATION (INFANT)

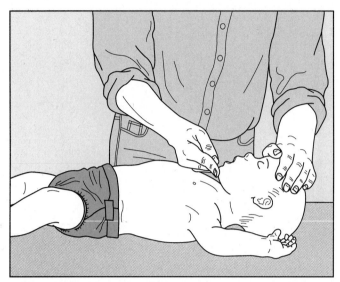

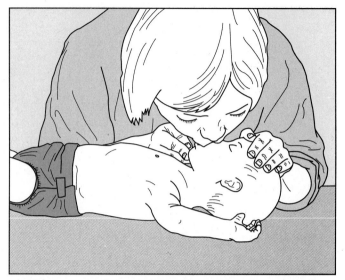

1 **Opening the airway.** Immediately have someone call for emergency help, then monitor the infant's vital life signs *(page 19)*. If the infant is not breathing or his breathing is shallow or uneven, open his airway by gently lifting his chin and pushing down on his forehead *(above)*. **Caution:** Overextending the infant's neck can cause an injury. Drop the infant's lower jaw, opening his mouth. If there is an obstruction in the infant's mouth, carefully remove it *(page 21)*. Otherwise, check for breathing *(page 19)*. If there is still no breathing or the breathing is shallow or uneven, blow air into the infant's lungs *(step 2)*. Otherwise, place the infant in the recovery position *(page 22)*.

2 **Blowing air into the lungs.** Keep the infant's airway open, holding his lower jaw to keep his mouth open. Take a breath and press your open mouth over the infant's mouth and nose, forming a tight seal. Deliver the breath through the infant's mouth and nose slowly in one short blow *(above)*, without allowing air to flow out of his lungs. **Caution:** Do not deliver a full, deep breath to the infant; air may be forced into his stomach or burst his lungs. Take another breath and deliver it the same way. After delivering two breaths slowly, break contact with the infant, allowing air to flow out of his lungs. Take a deep breath and check for breathing *(step 3)*.

3 **Checking for breathing.** Keep the infant's airway open to check for breathing *(page 19)*, dropping his lower jaw to open his mouth *(left)*. If there is no breathing or the breathing is shallow or uneven, blow air into the infant's lungs again *(step 2)*. If there is still no breathing, assume that the infant has choked and treat him *(page 21)*. Otherwise, continue to blow air into the infant's lungs, delivering one short breath slowly every 3 seconds. When the infant can breathe on his own, place him in the recovery position *(page 22)*. Monitor the infant's vital life signs *(page 19)* until emergency help arrives.

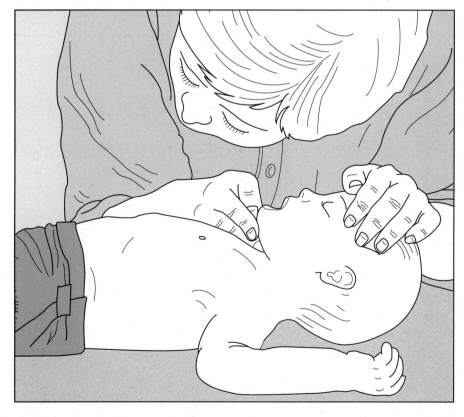

TREATING A CHOKING VICTIM (INFANT)

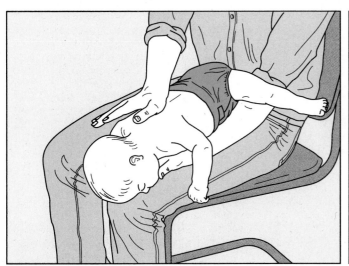

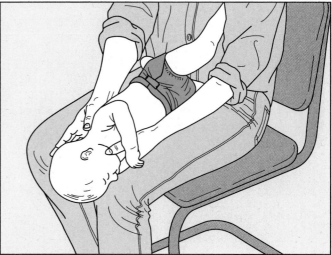

1 **Delivering back blows.** Immediately have someone call for emergency help. If the infant loses consciousness, act quickly to clear the obstruction *(step 3)*. Otherwise, place the infant face down on your thigh, using one hand to hold his chin and support his head lower than his feet. Using the heel of your other hand, deliver four firm blows to the infant's back between his shoulder blades *(above, left)*. Then, support the infant between your arms and with your hands to roll him over *(above, right)*, placing him face up on your thigh, again with his head lower than his feet. If the obstruction is removed, place the infant in the recovery position *(page 22)*. Otherwise, deliver chest thrusts *(step 2)*.

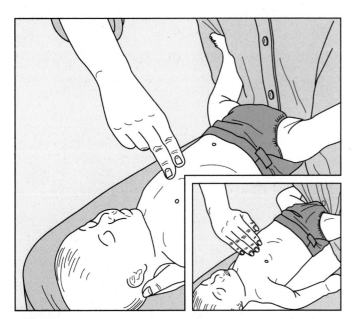

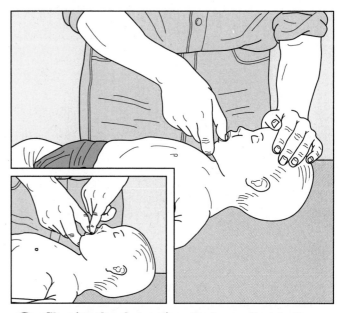

2 **Delivering chest thrusts.** To prepare to deliver chest thrusts, place three fingers of one hand against the midpoint of the infant's chest, the third finger between his nipples *(inset)*. Without moving your index and middle fingers, raise the third finger off the infant's chest. Deliver a chest thrust using only your index and middle fingers, pressing straight into the infant's chest cavity to a depth of 1/2 to 1 inch in one short quick, thrust *(above)*. Deliver three more short, quick thrusts about 1 second apart the same way. Then, check the infant's mouth for the obstruction and remove it *(step 3)*.

3 **Clearing the obstruction.** Gently open the infant's mouth with one hand, pressing his tongue down with your thumb and supporting his lower jaw with your index finger *(above)*. Looking into the infant's mouth, use the baby finger of the other hand to sweep in along one cheek, across the throat and back out along the other cheek *(inset)*, pulling out any obstruction. **Caution:** Do not make a blind finger sweep. When the obstruction is removed, monitor the infant's vital life signs *(page 19)*. Otherwise, continue to deliver back blows *(step 1)* and chest thrusts *(step 2)* until emergency help arrives.

PLACING A VICTIM IN THE RECOVERY POSITION

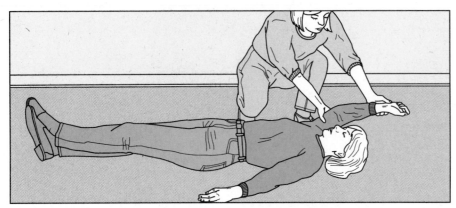

1 **Positioning the victim.** Immediately have someone call for emergency help, then monitor the victim's vital life signs *(page 12)*. **Caution:** If you suspect that the victim has suffered a spinal injury *(page 23)*, do not move him. Otherwise, place the victim on his back and loosen his clothing at the neck, chest and waist. Kneel beside the victim at his waist and cross his legs at the ankles, bringing the leg farthest from you over the leg closest to you. Take the victim's arm closest to you and extend it above his head *(left)*, then lay his other arm across his chest, bending it at the elbow.

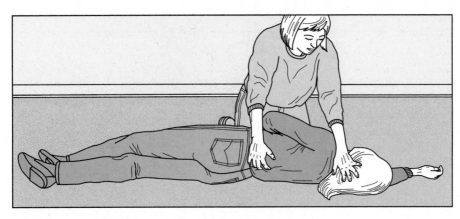

2 **Rolling the victim onto his side.** Place your knees as close as possible to the victim's chest and abdomen. Reach one hand across the victim and grip his shoulder firmly, then reach the other hand across him and slide it under his lower back; if necessary, grip a belt loop or other part of his clothing to hold him securely. Roll the victim toward you in one smooth motion, moving your hand from his shoulder to the back of his head to support his neck *(left)*. Stop rolling the victim when he is on his side, his chest and abdomen resting on your thighs.

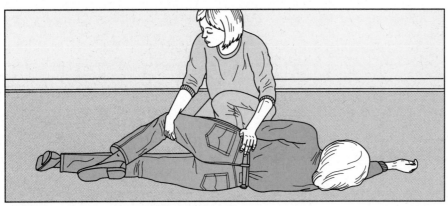

3 **Stabilizing the victim.** With one hand still on the back of the victim's head to support his neck, make sure that his head rests comfortably on his extended arm, cushioned by his shoulder; if necessary, raise his head slightly and reposition his extended arm to support it without it falling off. Placing one hand on the victim's lower back to support him, use your other hand to pull his upper leg toward you, bending it at the hip and the knee *(left)*; this position prevents the victim from rolling onto his chest. Carefully pull your knees away from the victim's chest and abdomen.

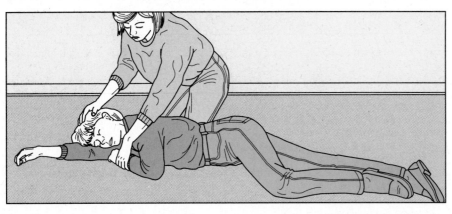

4 **Opening the victim's airway.** Supporting the victim's head on his extended arm, bend his other arm at the elbow and place it under him *(left)* to support his upper body; this position keeps the victim from rolling onto his face. Open the victim's airway by tilting his head back, gently lifting his chin and pushing his forehead; this action raises his lower jaw and draws his tongue away from the back of his throat.. Continue monitoring the victim's vital life signs *(page 12)* until emergency help arrives; if the victim is an infant *(page 19)*, keep him from rolling onto his back.

HANDLING A VICTIM OF A SPINAL INJURY

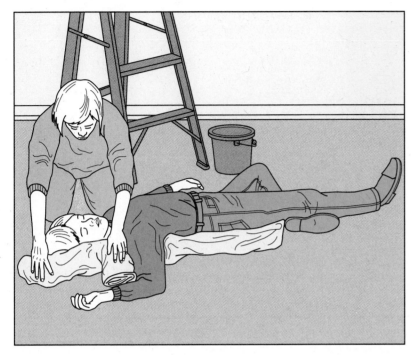

Treating a spinal injury. A spinal injury can be the result of a back, neck or head injury—caused by a fall or a blow, for example. If the victim has experienced a fall or a blow to his back, neck or head, you should suspect that he may have suffered a spinal injury. Signs of a spinal injury can include:

- Severe pain in the back, neck or head

- Tingling; loss of feeling or motion in the limbs

- Loss of bladder or bowel control

- Fluid or blood flowing from the ears or nose

- Loss of consciousness

   Immediately have someone call for emergency help, then monitor the victim's vital life signs *(page 12)*. **Caution:** Do not move the victim. Reassure the victim that emergency help is on the way, then immobilize his back, neck and head with blankets *(left)* or pillows. Keep the victim warm by covering him with a blanket and keep others away. Do not give the victim anything to eat or drink nor apply a hot-water bottle or heating pad.

HANDLING A VICTIM OF SHOCK

Identifying shock. Shock is the body's response to a failure of the circulatory system in providing sufficient blood to the brain or other vital organ. Shock can be provoked by a loss of blood or other fluid or by a heart attack, nerve injury, fright, pain or an allergic reaction. Some degree of shock—immediate or delayed—may accompany any injury or illness; its effects can be lessened if it is identified and action is taken quickly *(step right)*. Signs of shock can include:

- Restlessness or anxiety; lethargy, disorientation or confusion

- Pallor or bluish color of the skin

- Cold or clammy skin

- Profuse sweating

- Shallow, uneven or rapid breathing

- Weak, irregular or rapid pulse

- Extreme thirst

- Loss of consciousness

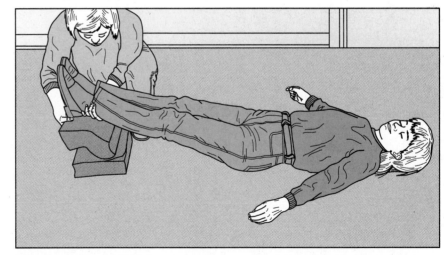

Treating a shock victim. Immediately have someone call for emergency help, then monitor the victim's vital life signs *(page 12)*. **Caution:** Do not move the victim if you suspect a spinal injury *(step above)* or he is in pain. Otherwise, if the victim is conscious, place him on his back with his head lower than his feet; elevate his legs and feet 8 to 12 inches with telephone books *(above)*, pillows or rolled-up blankets. Loosen the victim's clothing at his neck, chest and waist. Keep the victim warm by covering him with a blanket, but do not overheat him. Keep others from crowding around the victim. Do not give the victim anything to eat or drink; if he complains of thirst, moisten only his lips with water. Do not apply a hot-water bottle or heating pad to the victim.

HANDLING A VICTIM OF A HEART ATTACK

Identifying a heart attack. A heart attack is the result of a failure of the circulatory system in providing sufficient blood to the heart. The effects of a heart attack can be lessened if its signs are detected and action is taken quickly *(step right)*; half of the deaths attributed to heart attack are said to occur outside of a hospital setting within 2 hours of its onset. A heart attack can be difficult to detect, often identified mistakenly as heartburn or indigestion, for example. The victim of a heart attack may not seem ill—and even deny that he is suffering a heart attack. Be alert to the warning signs of a possible heart attack, especially if the victim has a history of heart problems:

- Tight or crushing pressure or pain across the chest that may radiate to the arms, neck, shoulders or jaw

- Heartburn or indigestion

- Labored breathing

- Weak or irregular pulse

- Cold, clammy skin

- Sweating

- Nausea

- Loss of consciousness

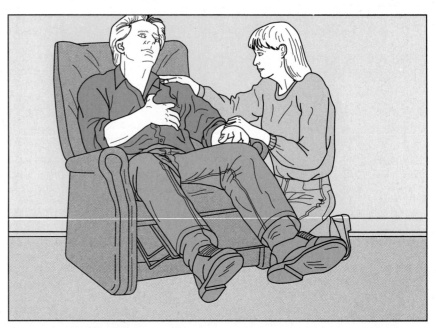

Treating a victim of a heart attack. Immediately have someone call for emergency help, then monitor the victim's vital life signs *(page 12)*. Reassure the victim that emergency help is on the way. If the victim is conscious, place him in a comfortable semi-sitting position, his head back and his feet up *(above)*. Loosen the victim's clothing at his neck, chest and waist. If the victim has a history of heart problems and is under a physician's supervision, help him to take any prescribed medication for his condition. Keep the victim warm by covering him with a blanket, but do not overheat him. Keep others from crowding around the victim. Do not give the victim anything to eat or drink; if he complains of thirst, moisten only his lips with water. Do not apply a hot-water bottle or heating pad to the victim.

HANDLING A VICTIM OF A STROKE

Identifying and treating a stroke. A stroke typically occurs when an artery of the brain ruptures, leading to internal bleeding, or when there is a blockage of an artery to the brain, interfering with the blood circulation to it. The signs and effects of a stroke can vary depending on the part of the brain that is affected; they can also range in degree and duration, sometimes passing quickly and recurring. Usually, however, a stroke can be characterized by its sudden onset. Be alert to the warning signs of a possible stroke, especially if the victim is more than 50 years old or suffers from high blood pressure:

- Disorientation, dizziness or confusion; a change of moods or shift of disposition

- Weakness, numbness, tingling sensations or paralysis on one side of the body—typically the face, an arm or a leg

- Headache; ringing in the ears

- Difficulty in speaking; slurred speech or garbled words

- Labored breathing

- Weak or irregular pulse

- Difficulty in swallowing

- Loss of bladder or bowel control

- Loss of consciousness

To treat the victim of a stroke, immediately have someone call for emergency help, then monitor his vital life signs *(page 12)*. Reassure the victim that emergency help is on the way. If the victim is conscious, place him in a comfortable semi-sitting position, his head back and his feet up. Loosen the victim's clothing at his neck, chest and waist; keep others from crowding around him. Do not give the victim anything to eat or drink; if he complains of thirst, moisten only his lips with water. If the victim vomits or loses consciousness, place him in the recovery position *(page 22)* on his affected side.

HANDLING A VICTIM OF AN ALLERGIC REACTION

Identifying and treating an allergic reaction. An allergic reaction is the body's response to exposure to an allergen—typically a food, a type of medication or the venom of an insect sting or bite. The signs and effects of an allergic reaction may vary and can be severe—in some instances, even fatal. A person vulnerable to a severe allergic reaction should wear medical identification, warning others of his condition *(page 9).*

Usually, exposure to an allergen provokes an allergic reaction in the victim within minutes. Be alert to the warning signs of a possible severe allergic reaction, especially if the victim has a history of allergy problems:

- Physical weakness or pain

- Pallor or discoloration of the skin; itchy rash or hives

- Swelling, especially around the eyes, lips, tongue or throat

- Labored breathing

- Weak, irregular or rapid pulse

- Profuse sweating

- Difficulty in swallowing

- Shock *(page 23)*

- Loss of consciousness

To treat the victim of a severe allergic reaction, immediately have someone call for emergency help, then monitor his vital life signs *(page 12).* Reassure the victim that emergency help is on the way and loosen his clothing at his neck, chest and waist; check his neck and wrist for medical identification. If the victim has a history of allergy problems and is under a physician's supervision, help him to take any prescribed medication for his condition. Keep the victim calm and comfortable; keep others away. If the victim loses consciousness, place him in the recovery position *(page 22).*

HANDLING A VICTIM OF A DIABETIC EMERGENCY

Identifying a diabetic emergency.
Diabetes occurs when the body lacks enough insulin for its cells to use the sugar in the blood. Two types of emergencies can arise: insulin shock from too little sugar; diabetic coma from too much sugar (and too little insulin). The type of emergency can be difficult to identify, but quick action can lessen its effects *(step right).* A diagnosed diabetic should wear medical identification, warning others of his condition *(page 9).*

Insulin shock usually is rapid in onset; it can be due to excess medication, insufficient food, strenuous physical activity or emotional stress. Be alert to the warning signs:

- Uneven or rapid breathing

- Rapid or irregular pulse

- Dizziness or physical weakness

- Profuse sweating

- Headache or vision difficulty

- Numbness of the hands or feet

- Loss of consciousness

Diabetic coma typically develops slowly; it can be due to insufficient medication, excess of sugar foods, emotional stress or infection. The signs to watch for include: drowsiness; deep, rapid breathing; thirst and dehydration; fever; and loss of consciousness.

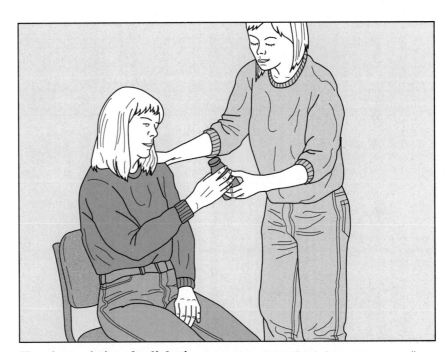

Treating a victim of a diabetic emergency. Immediately have someone call for emergency help, then monitor the victim's vital life signs *(page 12).* Reassure the victim that emergency help is on the way, checking his neck and wrist for medical identification. If the victim is conscious, place him in a comfortable sitting position and give him sugar—a fruit juice *(above),* soda pop or candy bar, for example. (Sugar helps the victim of insulin shock and does not harm the victim of diabetic coma.)
Caution: If the victim is a diagnosed diabetic, help him to take any prescribed medication for his condition only if diabetic coma is a certainty. If the victim loses consciousness, place him in the recovery position *(page 22)* and do not give him anything to eat or drink or any medication.

HANDLING A VICTIM EXPOSED TO LOW TEMPERATURE

Preventing frostbite and hypothermia. Unprotected skin exposed to extreme cold and high wind may become numb and white, symptoms of frostbite; the nose, ears, face, hands and feet are especially susceptible. Hypothermia is caused by prolonged exposure to cold; its victim can have a body temperature below 95° Fahrenheit and not shiver, as well as slowed, shallow or uneven breathing and a slow, weak or irregular pulse. Quick action can reduce the effects of frostbite and hypothermia *(step right)*; precautions during a cold snap or extremely low temperature can prevent them:

- Drink plenty of warm liquids to help maintain your body's temperature.

- Eat heavy meals of hot food.

- Keep out of direct exposure to the cold; if possible, stay indoors in a warm room.

- If you must venture outdoors, stay out of the wind and keep dry.

- Dress properly for cold weather, wearing clothing of heavy material that is dark-colored to help retain heat.

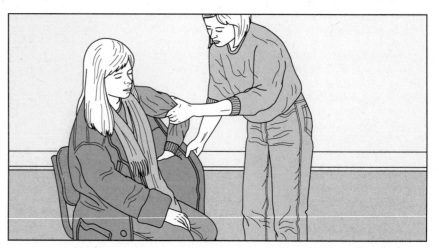

Treating a victim of cold exposure. Move the victim indoors, remove any wet clothing *(above)* and replace it with warm, dry clothing or blankets. If you suspect hypothermia or severe frostbite, immediately have someone call for emergency help, then monitor the victim's vital life signs *(page 12)*; also check his temperature *(page 114)*. Do not give the victim anything to eat or drink. Gradually warm the victim, focusing on areas of the body where heat loss is greatest: the head, neck, chest, armpits and groin. For areas of the body where there is frostbite, soak the skin with tepid water; do not apply hot water or direct heat. **Caution:** Do not rub frostbitten skin; crystallized moisture in it can cause severe injury. If the victim loses consciousness, place him in the recovery position *(page 22)*.

HANDLING A VICTIM EXPOSED TO HIGH TEMPERATURE

Preventing heat stroke. Heat stroke results from the body's inability to regulate its temperature during exposure to extreme heat. Sweating mechanisms that normally cool the body stop functioning as fluids are depleted, causing a rapid rise in temperature, muscular pains, cramps or spasms, and exhaustion. Quick action can reduce the effects of heat stroke *(step right)*; precautions during a heat wave or extremely high temperature can prevent it:

- Drink liquids to replenish body fluids lost by sweating—about 10 ounces of water every 15 minutes in extreme conditions.

- Keep out of direct exposure to the sun; if possible, stay indoors in an air-conditioned or well-ventilated, cool room.

- If you must go outdoors, stay in the shade. Wear a hat to protect your head from the sun, and clothing of light material that is light-colored to help reflect heat and sunlight.

- Eat frequent, small, light meals of cold food; avoid drinking alcohol.

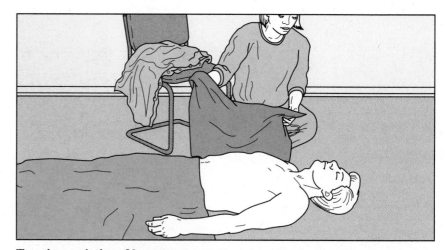

Treating a victim of heat exposure. Have the victim lie down in a cool place, elevating his feet and legs. Remove the victim's excess clothing and cover him with sheets soaked in cool water *(above)*. If you suspect heat stroke, immediately have someone call for emergency help, then monitor the victim's vital life signs *(page 12)*; also check his temperature *(page 114)*. Gradually cool the victim, focusing on areas of the body where heat is greatest: the head, neck, chest, armpits and groin. If the victim is conscious, give him plenty of cool water to drink and a cool bath. If the victim loses consciousness, place him in the recovery position *(page 22)*.

HANDLING A VICTIM OF A BURN

Identifying a burn. A burn is an injury to the skin tissue that may result from exposure to heat, a chemical, the sun, a hot liquid or steam, electrical current or lightning. The severity of a burn depends on the surface area and depth of the injury: a first-degree burn may provoke reddening of the skin; a second-degree burn may cause the skin to turn red and blister; a third-degree burn may result in dry, pale-white skin or brown, charred skin. By acting quickly, the pain and scarring of a burn can be lessened *(step right)*; treat it following the precautions listed below:

- Seek emergency help for any burn that is to the victim's face or genitals or that is larger in size than his hand.

- Remove the victim's clothing, jewelry and footwear before any swelling begins; leave in place any clothing adhered to the burn.

- Do not breathe on or touch the burn.

- Do not apply any antiseptic spray or ointment to the burn; never apply butter, margarine or oil.

- Do not apply a neutralizer such as vinegar, baking soda or alcohol to a chemical burn.

- Never break any blisters of the burn.

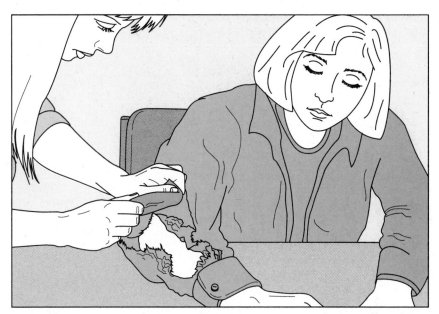

Treating a victim of a burn. If the burn is severe, immediately have someone call for emergency help, then monitor the victim's vital life signs *(page 12)*. Gently remove the victim's clothing from the burn; do not try to remove clothing adhered to it. Take off the victim's jewelry and footwear. Cover the burn lightly with a dry, sterile, gauze dressing *(above)* and elevate it above the level of the heart, if possible. Check the victim for signs of shock *(page 23)*. If the victim loses consciousness, place him in the recovery position *(page 22)*. If the burn is not severe, flush it for at least 10 to 15 minutes with a gentle flow of cool water from a faucet or garden hose, then bandage it with a sterile gauze dressing.

HANDLING A VICTIM OF ELECTRICAL SHOCK

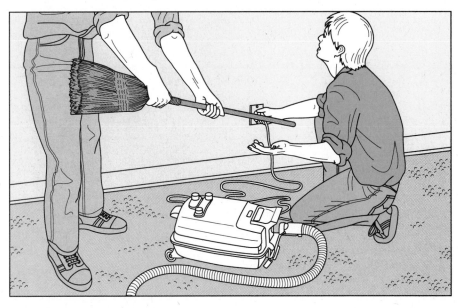

Treating a victim of electrical shock. A person who contacts live electrical current is usually thrown back from the source; sometimes, however, muscles contract involuntarily around the source, immobilizing the victim. **Caution:** Do not touch the victim or the source of electrical current. Immediately stop the flow of electricity by shutting off the power at the main circuit breaker, main fuse block or service disconnect breaker. If the power cannot be shut off immediately, use a dry wooden implement such as a broom handle, chair or board to knock the victim free of the source of electrical current *(left)*. Immediately have someone call for emergency help, then monitor the victim's vital life signs *(page 12)*. **Caution:** If you suspect a spinal injury *(page 23)*, do not move the victim. Otherwise, place the victim in the recovery position *(page 22)*.

HANDLING A VICTIM OF INGESTED POISON

Identifying ingested poisoning. Ingested poisoning is usually accidental or due to carelessness, but may be the result of an attempted suicide. The effects of ingested poisoning can be lessened if quick action is taken *(step right)* as soon as its symptoms are detected.

However, the symptoms of ingested poisoning can be difficult to detect. A child under the age of 6 is the most likely victim of ingested poisoning. If you suspect a child is the victim of ingested poisoning, ask him to show you the product he swallowed.

Be alert to the warning signs of a possible ingested poisoning that are listed below and take precautions to prevent an accidental ingested poisoning *(step below)*:

- Unusual breath odor

- Discoloration of the lips or mouth

- Dilated pupils

- Hot, dry skin

- Rapid, shallow or uneven breathing

- Rapid, weak or irregular pulse

- Lethargy or bizarre behavior

- Nausea, abdominal cramps or vomiting

- Loss of consciousness

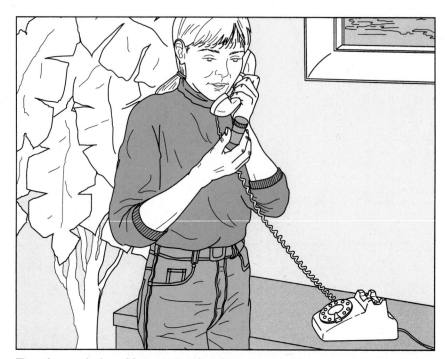

Treating a victim of ingested poisoning. Immediately have someone call for emergency help, telephoning the local poison control center or hospital emergency room; provide information on the type and amount of poison ingested *(above)*, as well as the victim's age and weight. Monitor the victim's vital life signs *(page 12)*, removing any foreign substance from his mouth. **Caution:** Do not give the victim anything to eat or drink or induce vomiting unless you are advised by a medical professional. If you are advised to induce vomiting, give the victim syrup of ipecac or glasses of warm water; or, instruct him to tickle the back of his throat with his finger. If the victim vomits or loses consciousness, place him in the recovery position *(page 22)*.

PREVENTING INGESTED POISONING

- To help childproof your home, install locks on the doors of all cupboards, cabinets and closets and all drawers containing medication or potentially-harmful household products.

- Keep all medication and all potentially-harmful household products well out of the reach of children; do not store them under sinks or in other easily-accessible places.

- Keep medication and household products in their original containers and do not remove the labels or instructions. Never transfer a medication or household product to a food or drink container.

- Carefully read the label on a medication before taking or administering it and follow the instructions exactly, paying close attention to all warning and caution statements.

- Do not take or administer medication in a darkened room without having first read the label on it and ensuring that the dosage has been correctly measured.

- Avoid telling a child that a medication tastes like candy.

- Never drink alcohol if you are taking a prescription medication.

- Administer a prescription medication only to the person named on its label; do not administer it to another person.

- Always replace the safety cap on a container. Put a medication or household product away safely as soon as you are finished with it; do not leave it out and unattended.

- Keep a bottle of syrup of ipecac on hand in the home; use it to induce vomiting only when instructed by a medical professional.

- To reduce the risk of an accidental ingested poisoning, avoid having unnecessary or seldom-needed medication and potentially-harmful household products on hand in the home; buy a product only in the volume that you need for immediate use and safely dispose of any that is left over.

TRANSPORTING A CONSCIOUS VICTIM

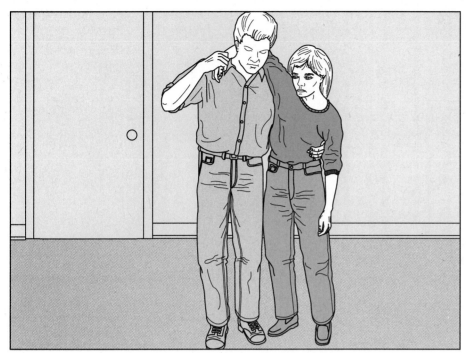

Moving a victim by yourself. Under certain conditions, a victim may need to be moved to a different location; if possible, move him with a helper *(step below)*. **Caution:** Do not move the victim if you suspect that he has suffered a spinal injury *(page 23)*, broken bone or other immobilizing injury. To move the victim by yourself, make use of your body as a crutch for him. Support the victim by taking one of his arms and draping it over your shoulder, then wrap your other arm around his waist. Have the victim lean against you to help carry his weight and slowly move forward *(left)*, taking short, smooth steps; lead with your foot that is farthest from the victim, then bring your other foot up to it. If the victim complains of pain, do not attempt to move him. Otherwise, continue until you reach your destination, then help the victim to position himself comfortably.

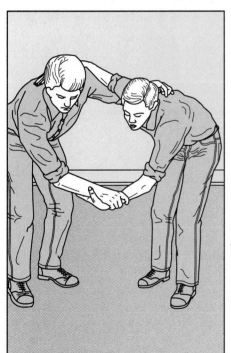
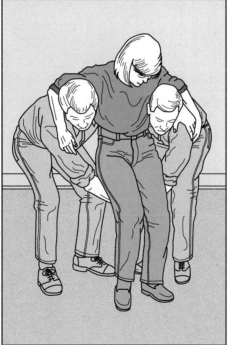
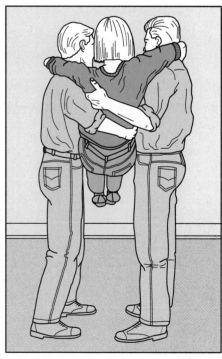

Moving a victim with a helper. Under certain conditions, a victim may need to be moved to a different location; if it is not possible to move him with a helper, move him by yourself *(step above)*. **Caution:** Do not move the victim if you suspect that he has suffered a spinal injury *(page 23)*, broken bone or other immobilizing injury. To move the victim with a helper, use a two-handed seat carry. Make a seat for the victim with your helper by placing opposite arms around each other's shoulders and firmly gripping each other's other arm firmly at the wrist *(above, left)*. Bend down at the knees until you are low enough for the victim to seat himself on your interlocked arms with his arms wrapped around your shoulders *(above, center)*, then use your other arms to support his back as you stand straight up *(above, right)*. Slowly move forward with your helper, taking short, smooth steps; lead with your feet that are farthest from the victim, then bring your other feet up to them. If the victim complains of pain, do not attempt to move him. Otherwise, continue until you reach your destination, then help the victim to position himself comfortably.

YOUR BODY

Fortunately, life-threatening medical illness is a rare occurrence for most families. Few families, however, can go a year without some type of minor injury, ache or pain, or infection—resulting in a cold, influenza, or a bout of vomiting or diarrhea. Digestive upsets due to stress, overeating or infection often cause a few sleepless nights. Minor accidents leading to cuts, bruises, splinters or sprains can seem to be weekly hazards of an active family life. And any medical problem, no matter how insignificant it turns out to be, can cause distress and worry as well as a disruption of daily routines.

Most minor health problems faced by the average family can be handled effectively at home; and with the prompt recognition and proper treatment of a minor health problem, the development of a serious medical disorder can often be averted. Every family should be familiar with the signs and symptoms of a possible health problem with each system of the body. Use the illustrations provided on page 31 to identify each major system of the body and for the first page of the chapter in this book devoted to it. Ensure that you and the other members of your family can correctly recognize and treat a minor health problem with any system of the body—and know when to consult a physician about the signs or symptoms of a potentially-serious disorder.

Prepare yourself to handle any medical crisis that may occur at home by studying the information presented in the Emergency Guide *(page 8)*; this chapter provides step-by-step instructions for dealing with typical life-threatening emergencies. Refer to the chapter entitled Equipment & Techniques *(page 110)* for the basic medical equipment to keep on hand at home and for techniques that can be useful in caring at home for a family member who is ill or recuperating from an illness.

Naturally, the best way for you and the other members of your family to handle medical problems is to maintain good health, adopting proper preventive-health practices. The health tips at right provide basic guidelines for maintaining your overall physical and mental health, referring you within this chapter and elsewhere in the book for more detailed information. For the typical family, there is a short list of health DOs: maintaining a well-balanced diet *(page 34)*, exercising regularly *(page 32)* and keeping a healthy home environment *(page 36)*. And for every family, the list of health DON'Ts should include: any abuse of alcohol *(page 35)* and cigarette smoking *(page 36)*.

Never ignore any sign or symptom of a possible medical problem or illness. For any uncertainty about the health of yourself or another family member, do not hesitate to call for help; medical professionals are available to answer your questions about symptoms and treatments. Post the telephone numbers for your physician, local hospital emergency room, ambulance and pharmacy near each telephone of your household; in most regions, dial 911 in the event of any life-threatening emergency.

HEALTH TIPS

1. Exercise regularly to maintain your overall physical and mental health as well as to prevent medical problems and illness; ensure that you take the steps necessary to exercise properly in order to prevent injury *(page 32)*.

2. To help ensure good mental health, build good physical health by exercising regularly, eating properly and getting plenty of rest and sleep *(page 33)*.

3. Learn to recognize and minimize the symptoms of stress *(page 33)* in order to maintain a healthy emotional life and prevent the physical strain that can lead to illness.

4. Maintain a balanced diet *(page 34)* to ensure that your body has a regular supply of all the nutrients it requires.

5. Maintain a body weight within an acceptable range *(page 35)* to minimize stress on the heart, lungs and muscles that can lead to chronic disease.

6. Familiarize yourself with the harmful physical effects of excessive alcohol; keep consumption moderate *(page 35)*.

7. Be aware of the life-threatening health risks posed by smoking cigarettes; realize the health benefits of stopping the habit, even for a long-time cigarette smoker *(page 36)*.

8. Minimize the health risks to you and your family from indoor pollutants by taking steps to reduce exposure to toxic substances in the home *(page 36)*.

9. Learn to recognize the early warning signs of illness *(page 37)*. Never hesitate to consult a medical professional about any symptom that worries you or any problem that you doubt your ability to manage.

10. Ensure that you and the other members of your family understand the importance of monitoring the body for unusual or persisting changes that may indicate a serious disorder such as cancer *(page 37)*.

11. Carefully follow the physician's directions to use any medication for an illness; use the amount specified at the prescribed times and report any side effect to the physician.

12. Avoid the use of any nonprescription medication to treat a medical problem unless your physician recommends it; a product may contain substances that can have negative side effects, especially if it is used carelessly.

13. Ensure that you and the other members of your family are familiar with the procedures for handling a life-threatening medical emergency in the home *(page 8)*.

14. Use basic home-care techniques for a family member who is ill or recuperating from an illness *(page 110)*, helping to ease the ordeal of illness for the patient—and you.

15. Establish an on-going relationship with your own physician. Always follow the schedule of routine medical checkups that is recommended for you by your physician.

BODY SYSTEMS

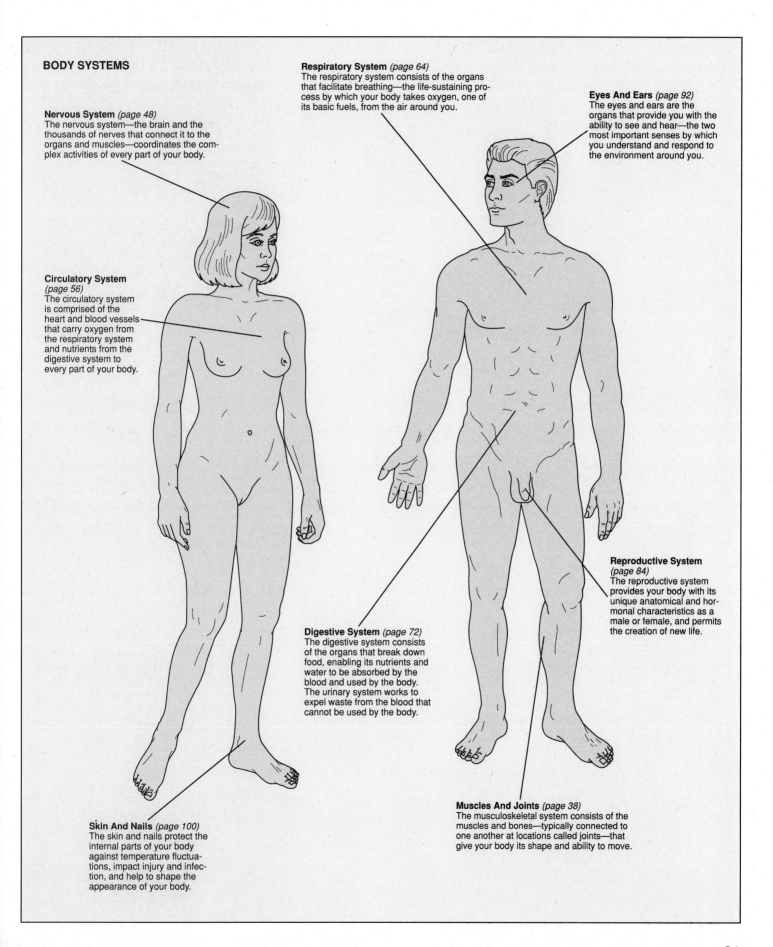

Respiratory System *(page 64)*
The respiratory system consists of the organs that facilitate breathing—the life-sustaining process by which your body takes oxygen, one of its basic fuels, from the air around you.

Eyes And Ears *(page 92)*
The eyes and ears are the organs that provide you with the ability to see and hear—the two most important senses by which you understand and respond to the environment around you.

Nervous System *(page 48)*
The nervous system—the brain and the thousands of nerves that connect it to the organs and muscles—coordinates the complex activities of every part of your body.

Circulatory System *(page 56)*
The circulatory system is comprised of the heart and blood vessels that carry oxygen from the respiratory system and nutrients from the digestive system to every part of your body.

Reproductive System *(page 84)*
The reproductive system provides your body with its unique anatomical and hormonal characteristics as a male or female, and permits the creation of new life.

Digestive System *(page 72)*
The digestive system consists of the organs that break down food, enabling its nutrients and water to be absorbed by the blood and used by the body. The urinary system works to expel waste from the blood that cannot be used by the body.

Skin And Nails *(page 100)*
The skin and nails protect the internal parts of your body against temperature fluctuations, impact injury and infection, and help to shape the appearance of your body.

Muscles And Joints *(page 38)*
The musculoskeletal system consists of the muscles and bones—typically connected to one another at locations called joints—that give your body its shape and ability to move.

EXERCISING REGULARLY

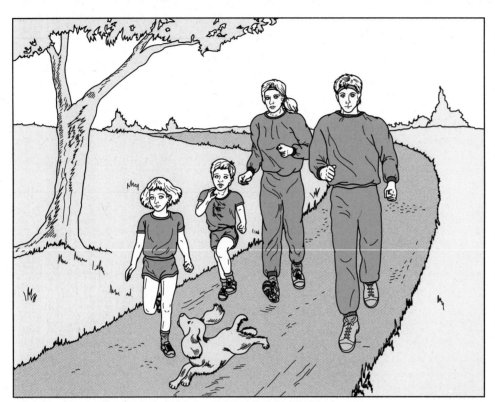

Understanding the benefits of exercise.

Many people associate exercise with tedious, gruelling and often painful physical exertion. Exercising properly *(step below)*, however, can be a relaxing and stimulating pastime—undertaken alone or as a social event with the family *(left)* or friends. Regardless of a person's age, regular, moderate exercise confers significant health benefits that can dramatically improve quality of life. Medical research indicates that a total weekly level of exercise equivalent to walking only 3 miles a day can significantly decrease the risk of heart disease by improving the ability of the heart and lungs to circulate blood to the organs, muscles and tissues of the body. Higher levels of exercise can further improve muscle tone and strength, but do not provide additional cardiovascular benefits. Other physical benefits of regular exercise include lower risk of calcium depletion that can weaken bones, elimination of unnecessary body fat, lower blood pressure and improved digestion. Exercise also has psychological benefits, including stress reduction, sleep enhancement, improved concentration and a heightened sense of well-being.

Exercising properly. While regular, moderate exercise can confer substantial physical and psychological benefits on most people, exercise that is sporadic, strenuous or done the wrong way can be harmful. Avoid being seduced into doing too much, too fast by the status or glamour associated with a popular fitness activity. The key to exercising properly is to find a type and level of activity that is beneficial to you alone.

Before taking up a rigorous activity, a person should consult his physician if he has not been physically active for a prolonged period of time; also if he is over 60 years of age, a smoker, overweight, or recuperating from an illness or surgery. A person should also consult a physician before undertaking an exercise program if he has a history of any of the following medical problems: back trouble, fainting spells, a chronic lung disease such as emphysema, a heart disorder, hypertension, diabetes or arthritis.

Refer to the guidelines below to plan a sensible exercise program that can provide the maximum of physical and psychological benefits—and prevent the risk of injury:

• Improve physical fitness gradually by finding daily routines and pastimes that increase your level of activity. To exercise your cardiovascular system, walk rather than drive, for instance.

• To undertake a new fitness activity regularly, choose one that you enjoy and can fit easily into your schedule. If an activity feels like punishment, you risk losing interest in it or doing it improperly.

• Undertake a new fitness activity intelligently. Learn all you need to know about the activity to do it properly, reading about it or receiving instruction on it from a qualified person, if necessary.

• Make a regular commitment to any fitness activity you choose. Schedule the activity each week at the same frequency and length of sessions, if possible always at the same times. Avoid the tendency to undertake an activity sporadically.

• Progress systematically with a fitness activity; do not attempt to work yourself into shape too rapidly. Start with just enough of the activity to become aware of mild physical strain, then increase the intensity of the activity gradually—never pushing yourself to the point of dizziness, exhaustion or pain.

• If you choose a competitive sport as a regular fitness activity, avoid the tendency to become overly competitive too quickly. Set your own personal goals and benchmarks; avoid the risk of personal injury from trying to outperform a competitor.

• Prevent injury during a fitness activity by wearing the safety equipment and clothing recommended for it. Maintain any safety equipment properly to prevent an accident while you are using it.

• To prevent indigestion and abdominal cramps, never undertake a strenuous fitness activity within 2 hours of a large meal.

• Avoid the risk of dehydration or heat exhaustion during any prolonged outdoor fitness activity by stopping at regular intervals to sip a non-alcoholic beverage.

• Do not undertake a fitness activity when you feel ill or are suffering from an illness—especially if you have a fever.

• Never undertake a fitness activity when you feel sleepy or fatigued; reduced mental alertness and physical coordination increase the risk of serious personal injury.

MAINTAINING MENTAL HEALTH

Keeping mentally alert. The cornerstone of good mental health is good physical health. A well-functioning body creates a positive self-image and sense of self-esteem. Good physical health also ensures that the brain itself is supplied with all the nutrients it requires to coordinate the complex functions of perception, judgment and analysis by which a person effectively manages life in a complex environment. As an example, approximately 20 percent of the oxygen absorbed by the blood from the respiratory system is required for use by the brain. A respiratory disorder that impairs the body's ability to get the oxygen it needs can seriously compromise the ability of the brain to function properly. There is no coincidence in the accompaniment of a typical physical illness with decreased mental functioning in the form of listlessness, reduced ability to concentrate and emotional distress. Maintain general mental health by taking the steps necessary to help guarantee overall physical health:

● **Exercise.** Undertake regular physical exercise *(page 32)* to activate the release of natural hormones within the brain that function to provide a sense of pleasure and reduce pain—what many athletes call a "natural high". Regular exercise in the form of cycling, jogging, skipping, swimming or walking can have a significant effect in reducing anxiety, tension and even depression. Improved cardiovascular health due to regular exercise means a steady, rich supply of oxygen for the brain that significantly improves alertness and powers of concentration.

● **Diet.** Maintain a proper diet *(page 34)* to ensure that the brain has a regular supply of the nutrients required by its tissues to function efficiently. For example, there is scientific evidence that suggests chronic overconsumption of high-fat foods may have a negative effect on powers of concentration—due to the increased need for oxygen-rich blood by the digestive system in doing the heavy work of breaking down these foods.. Other research indicates that carbohydrate foods with little or no protein may prompt the body to produce chemical substances that induce drowsiness. Meanwhile, still other research suggests that protein-rich foods stimulate the production of chemicals that heighten alertness.

● **Sleep.** Regular, proper rest and sleep each day are indispensable for proper mental functioning, permitting the body—and especially the brain—to continually rejuvenate itself for the busy work of the next day's activities. Occasional sleeplessness is normal, but chronic insomnia is a problem that requires the attention of a physician if it is not to provoke physical and mental problems. If necessary, take steps to minimize stress *(step below)* that interferes with proper rest and sleep. As well, regular exercise and the use of relaxation techniques *(page 46)* can help to ensure that the body gets the rest and the sleep it needs.

MINIMIZING STRESS

Understanding and managing stress. Stress is a complex set of body reactions that are triggered by the hypothalamus in the center portion of the brain. The hypothalamus is responsible for regulating the production and release of hormones by the body in response to stimuli entering the brain via the sensory organs of sight, sound and touch. In response to an external stimulus that induces fear, for example, the hypothalamus directs the adrenal gland to release adrenalin that speeds up the heart and readies the muscles for action.

● Consult a physician about a stress problem that interferes with your daily life; if necessary, seek long-term professional counseling about any cause of the problem.

● Identify the types of situations that induce stress, then minimize your exposure to them as much as possible in the future.

● When you begin to feel stress, stop what you are doing and take the time to analyze your reaction; ask yourself how you might react differently, then consciously try to react this way.

● Learn to handle anger effectively, avoiding the extremes of lashing out and ignoring it; try talking calmly about your anger, focusing on the emotions behind it.

● Learn to talk openly about problems with family members or friends; avoid hiding concerns or bottling them up.

Stress can become a problem for a person when the physical reactions of which it is comprised become severe and persistent. The symptoms of chronic stress can include tightness of the throat, sweating, tension headaches, fatigue, nausea or diarrhea. The typical procedure for managing chronic stress is to reduce exposure to the situations that trigger it, as well as to work at consciously altering the responses to it.

Refer to the guidelines presented below to help minimize the effects of a stress problem:

● Exercise regularly *(page 32)* to help you minimize stress—and respond with less of it in situations that can provoke it.

● To help prevent the development of a chronic stress problem, get plenty of regular rest and sleep.

● Avoid the energy-depleting effects of stress by eating regularly and properly *(page 34)*.

● Reduce physical tension due to stress with regular relaxation exercises *(page 46)*.

● Never use alcohol or a nonprescription medication such as a sleeping pill to try and treat a chronic stress problem.

● Learn to set healthy personal priorities; organize tasks into the essential, the important and the trivial, then forget about the trivial.

MAINTAINING A BALANCED DIET

Eating properly. Proper eating is a cornerstone of good health; it ensures that continuous supplies of essential nutrients pass from the digestive system into the bloodstream where they can be used by the hard-working organs and delicate tissues that need them. Ensure that you and your family plan a well-balanced diet *(step below)*, understanding its role in providing essential nutrients *(step right)*.

Proper eating helps to ensure that the body is supplied with the following essential nutrients:

• Protein—to build new organ and muscle tissue.

• Vitamins—to ensure the efficient operation of organ and muscle tissue.

• Minerals—to build bones and blood as well as produce enzymes and hormones.

• Starch and sugar—to provide quick energy to fuel metabolism.

• Fat—to provide concentrated energy to fuel metabolism and facilitate the absorption of vitamins.

• Fiber—to promote regular bowel movements and prevent digestive system disorders *(page 72)*.

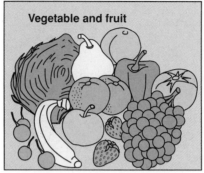
Vegetable and fruit

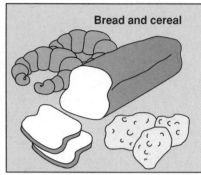
Bread and cereal

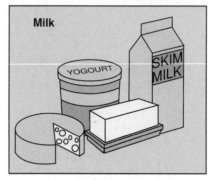
Milk

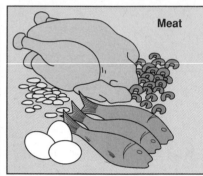
Meat

Understanding the role of a balanced diet. Maintaining a balanced diet ensures that the body has an adequate supply of the nutrients it needs to function properly. A balanced diet is one that includes foods from each of the four food groups *(above)*, as well as 6 to 8 glasses of water per day. In general, do not exclude a food group from your diet. If possible, choose a fresh rather than a processed food from a food group; processing can deprive a food of nutrients. Minimize consumption of any food that is high in fat, sugar, salt or caffeine.

FOOD GROUP	DAILY REQUIREMENT	FOOD	SERVING SIZE
Vegetable and fruit	4 servings; including at least 1 serving of food rich in vitamin C such as citrus fruit or yellow or dark green vegetable	Vegetable Potato Lettuce Salad, vegetable Salad, fruit Grapefruit Orange Melon	1 cup; sliced, raw 1 medium 1 wedge 1 medium bowl 1 cup; sliced, raw 1 medium 1 medium 1 medium
Bread and cereal	4 servings; including at least 1 serving of whole grain or enriched food	Bread Cereal, cooked Cereal, dry Rice Pasta	1 slice 3/4 to 1 cup 3/4 to 1 cup 3/4 to 1 cup 3/4 to 1 cup
Milk	2 to 4 servings; if lactose intolerance prevents milk consumption, consult a dietitian about alternative source of vitamin D and calcium	Milk Yogurt, plain Cheese, hard Cheese, spread Cheese, cottage Ice cream	1 cup 1 cup 1 1/4 oz. 2 oz. 2 cups 1 1/2 cups
Meat	2 to 4 servings; including at least 1 serving of plant-derived food such as beans, peas, nuts or seeds	Meat, cooked Poultry, cooked Fish, cooked Cheese, hard Cheese, cottage Eggs Dried beans or peas, cooked Nuts or seeds Peanut butter	2 to 3 oz. 2 to 3 oz. 2 to 3 oz. 2 to 3 oz. 1 cup 2 to 3 small 1 to 1 1/4 cups 3/4 to 1 cup 4 tablespoons

Planning a balanced diet. The daily diet advised for a typical healthy adult is 4 servings from the vegetable and fruit group, 4 servings from the bread and cereal group, 2 to 4 servings from the milk group and 2 to 4 servings from the meat group. Use the chart at left to identify common foods of a food group and the amount for a serving. For example, for a daily intake of 3 servings from the milk group, you may wish to take 1 cup of yogurt at breakfast, 1 cup of milk at lunch and 1 1/4 ounces of hard cheese at dinner.

Children and adults over the age of 65 require the same number of servings from each food group, but the size of each serving can be smaller. Children should eat full servings of calcium-rich foods from the milk group and iron-rich foods such as liver from the meat group. An elderly person not exposed to sunshine should eat a food that is high in vitamin D—butter from the milk food, or eggs or fatty fish from the meat group, for example.

Choose the required number of daily servings from each food group for a balanced diet, imaginatively combining them to create a tasty and nutritious menu for each meal. Take account of special needs when choosing foods; to control weight, for example, choose foods low in fat and sugar.

MAINTAINING PROPER BODY WEIGHT

Evaluating body weight. Maintaining body weight within an acceptable range is essential for good physical health. Too much or too little body weight can increase the risk of disease by putting stress on the heart and upsetting the nutrient balance of the blood. To determine if your body weight is a health risk, use the chart at right. Find the point indicating your height on the upper scale and the point indicating your body weight on the lower scale, then use a ruler to draw a straight line between the points and intersect the color-coded bar at the bottom of the chart. If the line intersects the bar section associated with little or no health risk, as in the example shown, ensure that you maintain your weight. If the line intersects a bar section associated with a slight health risk, eat less and exercise if your weight is too high; eat more and exercise if your weight is too low. If the line intersects the bar section associated with a significant health risk, consult a physician for a thorough medical examination and a safe, effective weight-loss program.

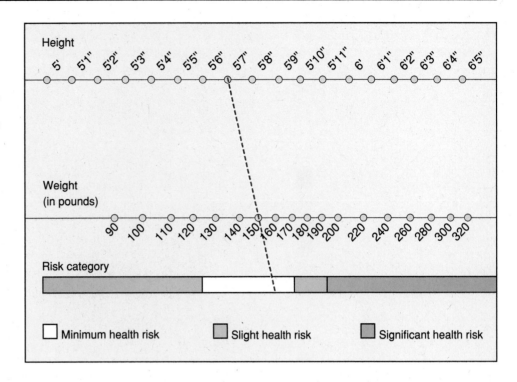

MINIMIZING ALCOHOL CONSUMPTION

Understanding the effects of alcohol. Food and water are essential for the body to function properly; alcohol, however, serves no nutritional benefit. Although moderate alcohol consumption is socially condoned and can be associated with pleasant sensations, chronic or excessive consumption of alcohol poses serious risks to physical and mental health. Temperance is essential *(step right)*, especially when driving a vehicle. For some individuals, as little as one drink can raise the blood alcohol content to a level that impairs functioning—or at which it is illegal to drive a vehicle.

Be aware of the health risks associated with chronic or excessive consumption of alcohol; in particular, educate children about the dangers:

• Liver disease—alcohol can destroy the liver tissue that helps to filter it out of the blood.

• Heart disease—alcohol can break down the tissue of the heart and promote clogging of the arteries, restricting the circulation of blood.

• Reduced immunity to infection—alcohol interferes with the production of white blood cells.

• Digestive disorders such as peptic ulcers—alcohol can damage the lining of the stomach.

• Birth defects—alcohol consumed during pregnancy can damage the fetus.

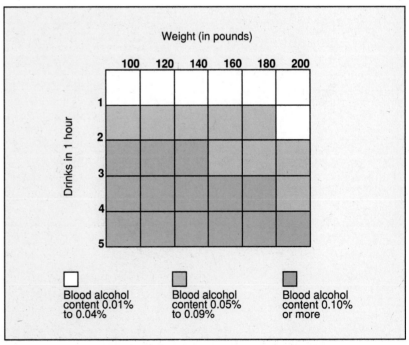

Drinking moderately. Refer to the chart above for the effects of alcohol consumption on blood alcohol content; a drink can be 12 ounces of beer, 5 ounces of wine or 1 1/4 ounces of 80-proof liquor. For most individuals, more than one drink in an hour achieves a blood alcohol content of 0.05 to 0.09 percent, a level that produces impairment of functioning—and at which it is illegal to operate a vehicle in many states. After two or three drinks in one hour, virtually all individuals achieve a blood alcohol content of 0.10 percent, a level that produces moderate to severe impairment of functioning. Keep your consumption of alcohol well below the level at which you risk impairment of your functioning; if you are operating a vehicle, well below the legal limit of impairment for driving.

ELIMINATING CIGARETTE CONSUMPTION

Understanding the risks of smoking. There is no secret about the risks of smoking cigarettes—the damage to health and the shortening of life expectancy. The more cigarettes a person smokes and the longer the period of time a person smokes cigarettes, the greater is the risk of disease and death. Be aware of the serious health risks of smoking cigarettes; in particular, teach children about the importance of avoiding the habit. If you smoke cigarettes, undertake every effort to quit the habit *(page 70)*.

The good news for smokers who quit the habit is the benefits to health and life expectancy, immediate and gradual—and an eventual reduction in the risk of disease and death to within the range of lifetime non-smokers. For example, a middle-aged adult who stops smoking cigarettes after many years of the habit can virtually eliminate his increased risk of death from a smoking-induced disease—in time to enjoy a full and healthy retirement. Consider the risks and benefits in making the decision to stop smoking:

Risks of 25-year smoking habit

- 10 times the risk of lung cancer than a non-smoker

- 6 to 15 times the risk of emphysema than a non-smoker

- 3 to 18 times the risk of larynx cancer than a non-smoker

- 3 to 10 times the risk of mouth cancer than a non-smoker

- 2 to 9 times the risk of esophagus cancer than a non-smoker

- 7 to 10 times the risk of bladder cancer than a non-smoker

- 2 to 5 times the risk of pancreas cancer than a non-smoker

Benefits of quitting 25-year smoking habit

- Gradually reduced risk; close to non-smoker after 15 years

- Reduced risk in 1 year; close to non-smoker after 10 years

- Gradually reduced risk; close to non-smoker after 10 years

- Gradually reduced risk; close to non-smoker after 15 years

- Gradually reduced risk; close to non-smoker after 10 years

- Gradually reduced risk; close to non-smoker after 7 years

- Gradually reduced risk; close to non-smoker in years

MAINTAINING A HEALTHY HOME ENVIRONMENT

Minimizing indoor pollution. The typical family spends a great deal of its time indoors. Within the home, however, there can be long-term health risks associated with exposure to dozens of chemicals, gases and dusts. Indoor pollution has been linked to a wide variety of adverse health effects—including headaches, respiratory problems, frequent colds and sore throats, chronic coughs, skin rashes, eye irritations, lethargy, dizziness and even memory lapses. Although proper ventilation can help to ensure good air quality within any home, the best strategy is to minimize the exposure of the family to as many indoor pollutants as possible. Follow the guidelines listed below to help you maintain a healthy environment within your home:

- Cigarette smoke contains over 1,500 known chemicals. Prohibit smoking in the home to prevent the pollution of indoor air.

- Avoid using commercial air-freshening products that may contain harmful chemicals; increase the circulation of air indoors instead by opening windows or using air conditioning.

- Install an exhaust fan for a gas range and use it when cooking with the range; a gas range may produce nitrogen dioxide and a host of other hydrocarbons.

- Have your home tested for radon gas seepage from the surrounding soil; if necessary, have your home professionally sealed against radon gas.

- Reduce your exposure to lead-containing airborne dust by vacuuming and washing household surfaces regularly; remove your shoes when you enter the house.

- Use sodium bicarbonate (baking soda) rather than a caustic commercial oven cleaner to scour an oven.

- Use a mild detergent rather than a cleaner containing a petroleum distillate to wash walls and floors.

- Wear rubber gloves to work with any product that contains harmful chemicals. Use any product that emits toxic vapors only in a well-ventilated area; always use any respiratory protection recommended by the product manufacturer.

- Avoid using a commercial shoe polish that contains methylene chloride, trichloroethylene or nitrobenzene.

- Hand-wash a fabric to try removing a stain before resorting to a potentially-harmful commercial spotter or dry cleaning fluid.

- Avoid using mothballs; instead, use a sachet containing dried lavender, rosemary, mint, dried tobacco, whole peppercorns and cedar chips soaked in cedar oil.

- Use isopropyl (rubbing) alcohol, soap or mild detergent for general cleaning jobs; avoid using a commercial disinfectant, especially if it contains phenol or cresol.

MONITORING HEALTH AT HOME

Recognizing the primary symptoms of illness. The body typically sends out early warning signals of impending illness. Unfortunately, these early warning signals often go unnoticed or unheeded until the full-blown illness develops. At the first sign of an impending illness, however, there are steps that can and should be taken to help prepare the body to fight it.

• **Fever.** Normal body temperature is 98.6° Fahrenheit. A raised temperature *(page 114)* is usually a sign that the body is fighting an infection. A person with a fever should stop routine activities and rest, using a nonprescription pain-reliever *(page 121)* to help reduce the fever. The person should be monitored for the development of secondary symptoms that more precisely indicate the nature of the illness, then treated specifically for it. Consult a physician immediately if a fever is extremely high, a secondary symptom appears to be serious, or a fever persists without secondary symptoms for more than 3 days.

• **Fatigue.** A lack of sleep or an inadequate or unbalanced diet can produce extreme tiredness—usually quickly rectified by sleeping properly and eating an adequate, balanced diet. Unexplained fatigue, however, is often a sign of an underlying physical or emotional disorder. A person who is chronically or recurrently listless or tired should be monitored for the development of secondary symptoms that more precisely indicate the nature of the illness, then treated specifically for it.

Immediate rest, adequate nutrition and generous fluid intake at the early stage of an illness can provide the body with the resources required to battle it—often preventing it from worsening. Be alert to the primary symptoms that precede virtually all illnesses, then take the necessary steps to strengthen the body and watch for the development of any secondary symptoms:

• **Appetite or weight loss.** An unexplained loss of weight or a sudden, marked loss of appetite is usually a sign of an illness at work in the body. A person who is chronically uninterested in food or who begins to lose weight without a change in diet or exercise patterns should be monitored for the development of secondary symptoms that more precisely indicate the nature of the illness, then treated specifically for it. In the absence of any secondary symptoms, consult a physician about any unexplained weight loss that continues for more than 1 month or appetite loss that lasts for more than 1 week.

• **Faintness.** Faintness or dizziness can result from prolonged exposure to a stuffy, poorly-ventilated environment, a sudden change of body position, or insufficient sleep or food. Recurrent, unexplained faintness or dizziness, however, can be a sign of an underlying physical disorder. A person who has frequent or persistent episodes of faintness or dizziness should be monitored for the development of secondary symptoms that more precisely indicate the nature of the illness, then treated specifically for it.

Detecting the early warning signs of cancer. Cancer is a devastating disease of the modern world, affecting not only the elderly, but people of all ages. Many forms of cancer, however, can be successfully treated if they are detected at an early stage. Regular, thorough medical examinations for all family members are excellent ways to help detect any problem at its early stage. There are also important steps that an individual can take to monitor himself for signs of cancer. Women, for example, should perform a self-

examination of the breasts monthly *(page 88)*; men should perform a self-examination of the testicles monthly *(page 89)*. All adults should monitor their bowel habits *(page 81)*. Every family member should understand the importance of a thorough knowledge of his own body—taking seriously any unusual, persistent or recurring change that occurs with it. While a bodily change often is the result of a minor, easily-treatable disorder, do not hesitate to consult a physician about any of the following:

• Unexplained, rapid weight loss

• Sudden appearance, growth or change in a mole on the skin

• Non-healing sore on the skin, especially of the face or a hand

• Unexplained, recurring fainting or dizzy spells

• Unexplained, recurring headaches

• Unexplained, recurring visual disturbances

• Episodes of vomiting with no preceding nausea

• Vomiting of blood

• Vomit of dried blood (consistency of coffee grounds)

• Unexplained, recurring shortness of breath

• Unexplained, persisting cough or hoarseness

• Coughing of blood

• Lump in the neck

• Lump or pain in a breast

• Unusual discharge from a nipple

• Unexplained, recurring abdominal pain

• Urine that is red or dark in color

• Stools that contain blood

• Unexplained, recurring constipation or diarrhea

• Recurring vaginal bleeding between periods or after intercourse

• Vaginal bleeding after menopause

• Lump or pain in a testicle

MUSCLES AND JOINTS

Your musculoskeletal system consists of the muscles and bones of your body—typically connected to one another at locations called joints. Together, the muscles, bones and joints give your body its external shape, house and protect its delicate internal organs, and, most importantly, permit you to move your body freely. The diagram on page 39 illustrates the complex network of muscles and bones that form the musculoskeletal system, and highlights the important hinge-like joints of the arms and legs that provide the body with its capacity for flexibility, mobility and dexterity.

Each joint is comprised of delicately-interlocked parts that work smoothly to permit it to move. A layer of cartilage acts as a shock absorber between the ends of two bones that form a joint. A ligament that connects the end of one bone to another permits movement while keeping the bones aligned. The ends of muscles are attached to the ends of the bones where they enter a joint—either directly or by means of a short tendon. The joint is filled with tiny sacs or bursa that lubricate the joint and permit movement without friction. Pain in a joint may result from a tearing, stretching or inflammation of any or all of the parts of it.

The musculoskeletal system of the average, healthy person develops few problems on its own, provided it is treated with a modicum of respect. Overexertion, stress, poor posture and accidents due to carelessness can all do damage to muscles, joints and bones, however. Similarly, the bones of the proverbial "couch potato" can become thin and brittle, the muscles can lose their strength and the ligaments can tighten, restricting movement of the joints. The list of health tips at right covers basic guidelines to keep the musculoskeletal system as strong and flexible as it needs to be to carry you through a lifetime of work and play.

The Troubleshooting Guide *(page 40)* puts procedures for everyday aches and pains of the muscles and joints at your fingertips, and refers you to pages 41 to 47 for more detailed informaion. Familiarize yourself with procedures for relieving a painful muscle cramp *(page 45)* and for treating a sprain *(page 42)*. For tired and sore muscles of the back, neck and shoulders, you can use relaxation exercises to relieve muscle tension *(page 46)* and prevent the development of serious problems. If you or a family member shows signs of developing a chronic joint disorder such as arthritis, you can take steps to manage it *(page 41)*. For techniques on handling a life-threatening emergency such as a suspected spinal injury, consult the Emergency Guide *(page 8)*. For basic techniques on caring for a family member who is ill or recuperating from an illness, consult the Equipment & Techniques chapter *(page 110)*.

If you must cope with a muscle or joint problem, do not hesistate to call for help; medical professionals can answer questions about symptoms and treatments. Post the telephone numbers for your physician, local hospital emergency room, ambulance and pharmacy near the telephone; in most regions, dial 911 in the event of a life-threatening emergency.

HEALTH TIPS

1. To strengthen your muscles, joints and bones, get plenty of exercise and fresh air—without overdoing it. Walk rather than drive, for example; or, take up a pastime such as swimming, cycling or gardening, choosing an activity to suit your tastes and physical strength.

2. To maintain healthy muscles, joints and bones, eat a diet rich in protein, calcium and vitamin D—a vitamin that helps the body absorb calcium. Consult a nutritionist to determine the levels you require and to plan an appropriate diet.

3. To maintain healthy muscles, joints and bones, sleep well every night. Reduce stress-related muscle tension by regularly doing relaxation exercises *(page 46)* or having a professional massage.

4. To prevent mishaps that can damage muscles, joints and bones, minimize the chance of a slip or a fall by maintaining a safe household. Keep floor and stair surfaces clutter-free. Use no-slip mats and handrails in bathtubs and shower stalls. Work carefully in high places and when using ladders.

5. To prevent serious damage to muscles, joints and bones from an accident, always wear a seat belt when riding in a car, a heavy-duty crash helmet when riding on a motorcycle and a light crash helmet when riding on a bicycle.

6. To prevent muscle and joint problems of the back, develop the habit of standing, sitting and sleeping with the correct posture. Always lift a heavy object properly *(page 44)*.

7. To prevent muscle and joint problems of the feet and ankles, care for and exercise the feet and ankles properly *(page 47)*. Always wear footwear that is appropriate for the activity; if you walk or jog, for example, a pair of proper shoes is a good investment.

8. To prevent muscle and joint problems, undertake any sport or fitness activity wisely. Select a physical activity appropriate for your age, size and abilities. Learn the rules for the activity and follow them. Warm up before and cool down after any strenuous activity. Always use the proper equipment, and wear the appropriate protective gear and clothing for the activity. Listen to your body; if an activity starts to hurt, stop.

9. Consult a physician about any potentially-serious symptom of a muscle, joint or bone problem such as: recurrent, persistent or severe pain or swelling; any loss of sensation or movement; or, any problem that interferes with or restricts the ability to use a muscle or joint.

10. Follow the physician's directions to use any prescription medication for a muscle or joint problem; use the amount specified at the prescribed times and report any side effect to the physician.

11. If you suffer from a chronic muscle or joint problem such as arthritis or if you are not normally physically active, consult a physician before undertaking a rigorous physical activity; if recommended, consult a physiotherapist about an exercise program to gradually increase your physical capacity.

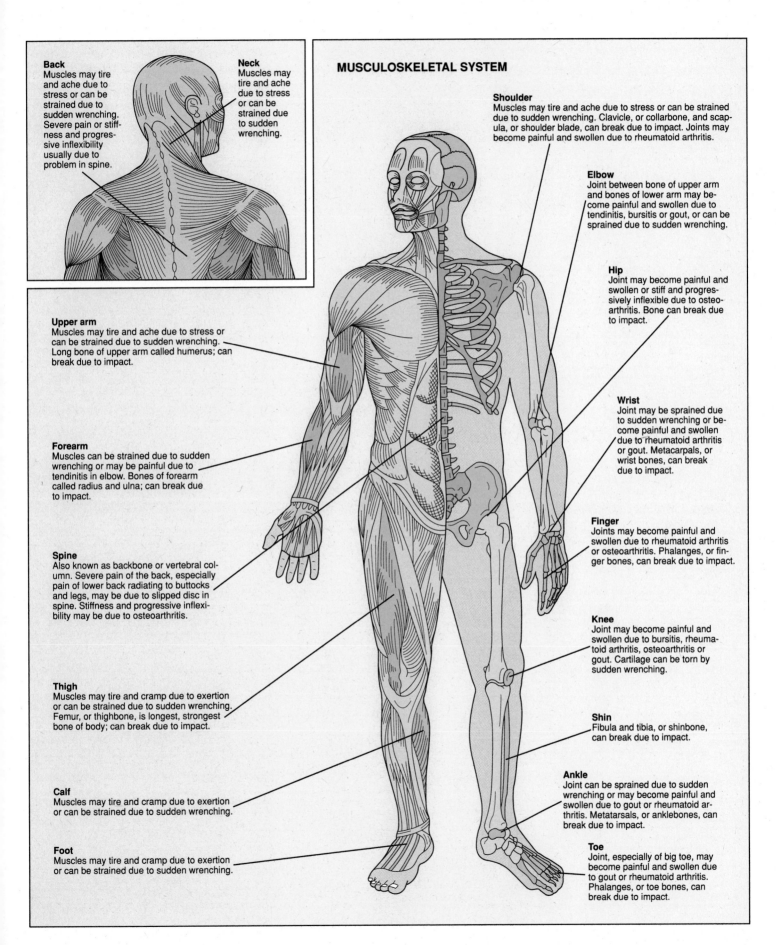

Back
Muscles may tire and ache due to stress or can be strained due to sudden wrenching. Severe pain or stiffness and progressive inflexibility usually due to problem in spine.

Neck
Muscles may tire and ache due to stress or can be strained due to sudden wrenching.

MUSCULOSKELETAL SYSTEM

Shoulder
Muscles may tire and ache due to stress or can be strained due to sudden wrenching. Clavicle, or collarbone, and scapula, or shoulder blade, can break due to impact. Joints may become painful and swollen due to rheumatoid arthritis.

Elbow
Joint between bone of upper arm and bones of lower arm may become painful and swollen due to tendinitis, bursitis or gout, or can be sprained due to sudden wrenching.

Hip
Joint may become painful and swollen or stiff and progressively inflexible due to osteoarthritis. Bone can break due to impact.

Wrist
Joint may be sprained due to sudden wrenching or become painful and swollen due to rheumatoid arthritis or gout. Metacarpals, or wrist bones, can break due to impact.

Finger
Joints may become painful and swollen due to rheumatoid arthritis or osteoarthritis. Phalanges, or finger bones, can break due to impact.

Knee
Joint may become painful and swollen due to bursitis, rheumatoid arthritis, osteoarthritis or gout. Cartilage can be torn by sudden wrenching.

Shin
Fibula and tibia, or shinbone, can break due to impact.

Ankle
Joint can be sprained due to sudden wrenching or may become painful and swollen due to gout or rheumatoid arthritis. Metatarsals, or anklebones, can break due to impact.

Toe
Joint, especially of big toe, may become painful and swollen due to gout or rheumatoid arthritis. Phalanges, or toe bones, can break due to impact.

Upper arm
Muscles may tire and ache due to stress or can be strained due to sudden wrenching. Long bone of upper arm called humerus; can break due to impact.

Forearm
Muscles can be strained due to sudden wrenching or may be painful due to tendinitis in elbow. Bones of forearm called radius and ulna; can break due to impact.

Spine
Also known as backbone or vertebral column. Severe pain of the back, especially pain of lower back radiating to buttocks and legs, may be due to slipped disc in spine. Stiffness and progressive inflexibility may be due to osteoarthritis.

Thigh
Muscles may tire and cramp due to exertion or can be strained due to sudden wrenching. Femur, or thighbone, is longest, strongest bone of body; can break due to impact.

Calf
Muscles may tire and cramp due to exertion or can be strained due to sudden wrenching.

Foot
Muscles may tire and cramp due to exertion or can be strained due to sudden wrenching.

TROUBLESHOOTING GUIDE

PROBLEM	PROCEDURE
Bone break, or cartilage or ligament tear suspected*: severe pain, swelling and bruising due to impact; injured area visibly misshapen or movement impossible	Seek emergency help ✚
	If necessary, use emergency first aid (p. 8)
Muscle tension*: periodic fatigue, soreness and stiffness of muscles due to stress	Use relaxation exercises to relieve muscle tension (p. 46)
	Prevent back problems by standing, sitting, lifting and sleeping properly (p. 44)
Muscle cramp*: sudden, painful spasm of muscle due to strenuous activity	Relieve muscle cramp (p. 45)
	Consult a physician if muscle cramps frequent
Muscle strain suspected*: rapid onset of pain and tenderness of muscle due to wrenching	Seek emergency help ✚ if pain severe, injured area visibly misshapen, or loss of sensation or movement experienced
	Treat muscle strain (p. 42)
	Consult a physician if pain or swelling lasts more than 3 days or muscle weakness or tenderness lasts more than 2 weeks
Joint sprain suspected*: rapid onset of pain, swelling and bruising of joint due to wrenching	Seek emergency help ✚ if pain severe, injured area visibly misshapen, or loss of sensation or movement experienced
	Treat joint sprain (p. 42)
	Consult a physician if pain or swelling lasts more than 3 days or joint weakness or tenderness lasts more than 2 weeks
Tendinitis suspected*: steady onset of pain and tenderness of joint due to prolonged overuse; pain may radiate out from joint	Relieve pain and swelling, and consult a physician to monitor and treat joint disorder (p. 41)
Bursitis suspected*: steady onset of pain, swelling and tenderness of joint due to prolonged overuse	Relieve pain and swelling, and consult a physician to monitor and treat joint disorder (p. 41)
Gout suspected*: general malaise, rapid onset of redness, pain, swelling and extreme tenderness of joint	Relieve pain and swelling, and consult a physician to monitor and treat joint disorder (p. 41)
Rheumatoid arthritis suspected*: general malaise, steady onset of redness, stiffness, pain (worst in morning) and swelling of joint	Relieve pain and swelling, and consult a physician to monitor and treat joint disorder (p. 41)
	If necessary, take steps to manage arthritic disorder (p. 41)
Osteoarthritis suspected*: aging; slow onset of decreasing flexibility, stiffness, aching and swelling of joint	Relieve pain and swelling, and consult a physician to monitor and treat joint disorder (p. 41)
	If necessary, take steps to manage arthritic disorder (p. 41)
Foot fatigue: periodic soreness and stiffness of feet and ankles	Prevent foot and ankle problems by caring for and exercising feet and ankles (p. 47)
Bunion suspected: slow onset of swelling of big toe joint; skin red, hard and tender; toe turns inward	Relieve pressure on bunion from shoes by using bunion pads available at a pharmacy
	Consult a physician to treat bunion
Heel spur suspected: painful, tender spot on heel; feels like bruise	Relieve pain as you would to treat a sprain or strain (p. 42)
	Consult a physician to treat heel spur

✚ Medical emergency

*PROBLEM	AREA MOST VULNERABLE
Bone break	Arm, finger, leg or toe
Cartilage or ligament tear	Elbow, wrist, knee or ankle
Muscle tension	Neck, shoulder or back
Muscle cramp	Thigh, calf or foot
Muscle strain	Neck, shoulder, back, upper arm, thigh or calf
Joint sprain	Elbow, wrist, finger, knee, ankle or toe
Tendinitis	Elbow, wrist, knee or ankle
Bursitis	Shoulder; also elbow, hip or knee
Gout	Big toe; also elbow, wrist, finger, knee or ankle
Rheumatoid arthritis	Wrist, finger, knee, ankle or toe
Osteoarthritis	Lower spine, knee or big toe; also hip or finger

MONITORING AND TREATING A JOINT DISORDER

Managing a joint disorder. Consult a physician about any gradual or sudden onset of pain, tenderness, inflammation, swelling or stiffness in a joint that is not due to an identifiable injury or overexertion. Rest and use the joint as little as possible. To relieve pain and swelling of the joint, use a nonprescription pain reliever *(page 121)* and administer cold treatments for 48 hours, then heat treatments.

• **Blood tests and X-rays.** If you suspect that a joint problem may be due to gout, osteoarthritis or rheumatoid arthritis, ask your physician to do a blood test to help rule out other infections or disorders that may be causing the symptoms. And for any of these suspected disorders or if you suspect tendinitis, talk to the physician about doing an X-ray of the affected joint to help determine the extent of the problem.

• **Prescription medications.** If the pain or swelling of a joint is severe, ask your physician about using a prescription medication. Follow the directions on the label of any prescription medication, using only the amount specified at exactly the prescribed times. Note any side effects of the medication or any change in how quickly or well it works and report the information to the physician.

• **Diet.** If you are overweight and you suspect that a joint problem is due to gout, osteoarthritis or rheumatoid arthritis, talk to your

For a cold treatment, apply an ice pack to the affected joint for 15 to 20 minutes at a time; for a heat treatment, apply a hot-water bottle to the affected joint for the same time interval. For additional relief to a joint of the arm, use an arm sling *(page 43)*. Refer to the guidelines below to talk to your physician about managing any acute or chronic joint disorder:

physician about a diet to reduce weight and minimize pressure on the affected joint or joints. If you suspect gout, also ask the physician about a diet to reduce the intake of foods that can cause a painful buildup of uric acids in the joints.

• **Physiotherapy.** If you suspect that a joint problem is due to tendinitis or to a chronic disorder such as osteoarthritis or rheumatoid arthritis, talk to your physician about using physiotherapy to prevent deterioration of the muscles surrounding the affected joint or joints. Then, find a physiotherapist who can design a program suited to your condition and activity level.

• **Surgery.** If you suspect that a joint problem is due to bursitis, osteoarthritis or rheumatoid arthritis—especially if there is severe pain or deterioration is rapid—talk to your physician about the possibility of eventual surgery that may help to restore use of the affected joint or joints.

MANAGING AN ARTHRITIC DISORDER

Living with arthritis. Millions of Americans are affected by some form of arthritis—whether rheumatoid arthritis, osteoarthritis or chronic gout. The first thing to do if you suspect arthritis is to embark on a proper, long-term course of identification and treatment to manage the symptoms of the disorder *(step above)*. And if you or a family member suffers from arthritis, take the steps neces-

• **Kitchen.** Store supplies on low, open shelves instead of high up in cupboards. Hang pots and utensils on pegboards at comfortable heights. Use light utensils with large, easy-to-hold handles. Sit on a chair or a stool rather than stand to work at a counter; install counters or tables at heights for sitting comfortably. Use light small appliances to minimize work—an electric knife, can opener or jar opener, for example.

• **Bathrooms.** Slide sponge hair rollers over the handles of toothbrushes and combs for an easy grip. Use low, open shelves for storage rather than vanity or medicine cabinets with doors. Make sure that the bathtub or shower stall has anti-slip decals or a good-quality rubber mat to reduce the chances of slipping or falling; install a handrail to make it easy to get into and out of the bathtub or shower, and keep a chair or stool nearby.

• **Doors and stairs.** Use a key holder with a large grip to insert and turn a key in a door lock easily. If stairs are a problem, install a ramp or have a staircase redesigned and fitted with shallower risers, wider treads and sturdy handrails.

sary to make your home environment manageable for someone with arthritis. While pharmacies and medical supply centers carry many commercial aids to assist arthritis sufferers in effectively performing routine tasks, refer to the guidelines below to troubleshoot and upgrade your home, making daily life as simple and comfortable as possible for an arthritis sufferer:

• **Workroom.** Use light tools with large handles. Wrap tool handles in cloth tape to ensure a secure grip. To minimize crouching or bending when working outdoors, use light, plastic tools; use gardening tools with long handles. Fit slip-on covers over pencils to make them easy to grip.

• **Bedroom closets.** To minimize the need to reach, install low shelves on which to arrange closet items. Install hooks and baskets on the back of the closet door for accessible storage spaces. To minimize the need to bend over, put shoes on racks or in hanging shoe bags rather than on the floor of the closet.

• **Clothing.** To make it easy to undo the zipper on an article of clothing, put an easy-to-grasp ring on the zipper. Replace difficult-to-manipulate zippers or buttons on articles of clothing with self-adhering nylon fasteners. To minimize the need to bend over, wear shoes that can be slipped on and off easily while standing or use a shoehorn with a long handle. Use elastic rather than nylon shoelaces in order to slip shoes on and off without undoing them. Use a long, hooked dowel for pulling on socks.

MUSCLES AND JOINTS

TREATING A SPRAIN OR STRAIN

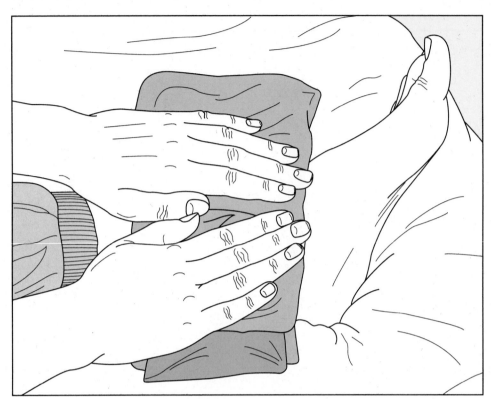

Relieving pain and swelling. To treat a sprained joint or a strained muscle, rest and use it as little as possible until any pain or swelling subsides—usually several days. To relieve pain and swelling of the sprain or strain, administer cold treatments for 48 hours, then heat treatments. Lie or sit in a position that minimizes discomfort and remove any jewelry, clothing or footwear from the injured area. For a cold treatment, apply an ice pack or a plastic bag of ice cubes wrapped in a towel *(left)* for 15 to 20 minutes. For a heat treatment, apply a hot-water bottle for the same time interval. For additional relief to a sprained ankle, use an ankle bandage *(step below)*; for a sprain or strain to the arm, use an arm sling *(page 43)*. To strengthen the joint or muscle before using it again, limber it up by gently moving it through its full range of motion without putting weight on it; once it is strong, increase the use of it gradually. Consult a physician if any pain or swelling persists after 3 days or if the joint or muscle is still weak or tender after 2 weeks.

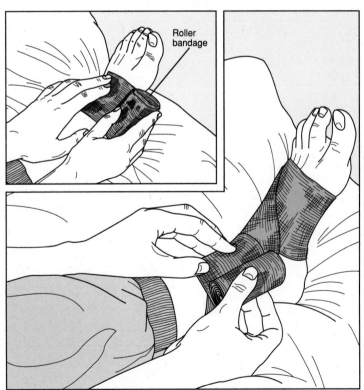

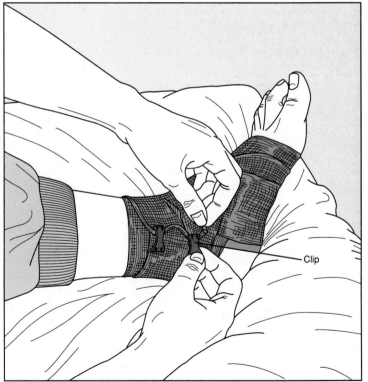

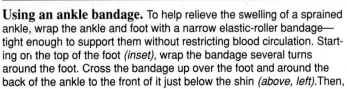

Using an ankle bandage. To help relieve the swelling of a sprained ankle, wrap the ankle and foot with a narrow elastic-roller bandage—tight enough to support them without restricting blood circulation. Starting on the top of the foot *(inset)*, wrap the bandage several turns around the foot. Cross the bandage up over the foot and around the back of the ankle to the front of it just below the shin *(above, left)*. Then,

cross the bandage back down over the foot and under it again to complete a figure-8 pattern. Continue the same way, wrapping the bandage up over the foot around the ankle, then back down over the foot and under it, overlapping each layer by 2/3 the bandage width. Finish wrapping the bandage with a turn around the ankle. Secure the loose end of the bandage to the wrapped part of it with bandage clips *(above, right)*.

USING AN ARM SLING

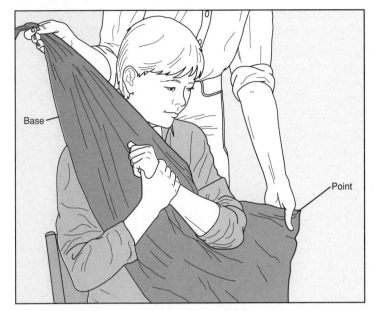

1 **Draping the bandage.** To temporarily immobilize a weak or injured arm, make an arm sling using a large triangular bandage. Have the person stand or sit upright and hold the injured arm diagonally across the chest in as high a position as is comfortable. Unfold the bandage and lay it on the person's lap, then draw it under the injured arm and across the chest. Hold the bandage by one end of its base over the shoulder of the uninjured arm and by its point below the elbow of the injured arm *(above)*.

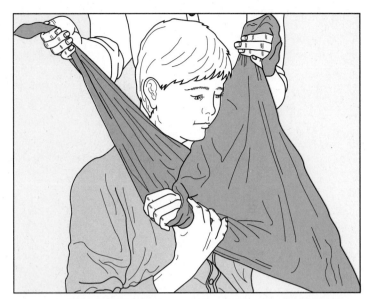

2 **Folding the bandage around the arm.** Fold the bandage carefully over the person's injured arm by drawing the other end of its base up to the shoulder of the injured arm. Then, gently adjust the position of the bandage *(above)* until the ends of its base meet behind the victim's neck and the hand of the injured arm is supported about 4 inches above the elbow of the uninjured arm. If the person complains of severe pain, do not continue; have the person stabilize the injured arm in as comfortable a position as possible and seek medical help for the arm injury.

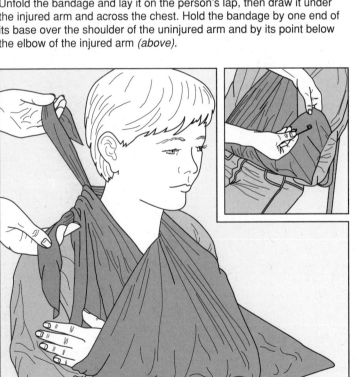

3 **Securing the sling.** With the person supporting the injured arm, secure the bandage at the side of the neck opposite the injury, tying the ends of its base into a knot *(above)* that can sit comfortably in the hollow of the shoulder. Smooth out the point of the bandage extending beyond the elbow of the injured arm and neatly fold it forward toward the elbow, then gently wrap it up over the upper arm. Secure the bandage with adhesive tape or a safety pin *(inset)*, taking care not to prick the upper arm.

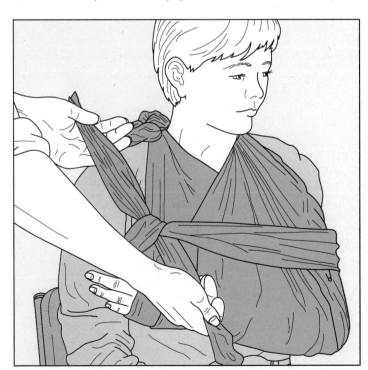

4 **Stabilizing the sling.** To immobilize the arm and hold it against the chest for additional support, make a swathe about 4 inches wide; fold a large triangular bandage into a strip or improvise using a strip from a towel, blanket or shirt. Wrap the swathe around the person just above the injured arm, passing over it and under the uninjured arm. To secure the swathe, tie its ends together into a knot on one side of the uninjured arm *(above)*. If necessary, seek medical help for the arm injury.

PREVENTING A BACK PROBLEM

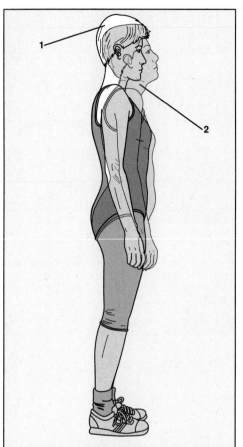

Standing properly. Familiarize yourself with the elements of good standing posture, then assess the elements of your posture as often as you can to develop the habit of standing properly. When you stand properly, you should be able to imagine that a line dropped from your earlobe can run just past the tip of your shoulder and continue down along the middle of your thigh, past the back of your knee to stop just in front of your ankle *(left, 1)*. Avoid standing with the chin up, the shoulders stooped, the abdomen thrust forward or the buttocks thrust back, any of which creates a sway-backed posture *(left, 2)*; also avoid standing with the shoulders pulled back and the chest thrust forward. If you must stand for a long period, alternately elevate each foot to rest it on a raised surface such as a stool or chair rung to reduce strain on the back.

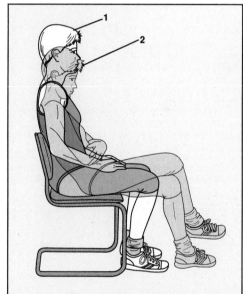

Sitting properly. Because sitting is normally associated with relaxing, it is easy to forget that sitting actually places great stress on the back. Whenever you sit, choose a sturdy chair with a back that provides full support for your lower back; ensure that the seat is low enough to keep your knees at or above the level of your hips when you sit. Sit properly to minimize stress on your back and prevent back problems. Keep your back straight against the back of the chair, relax your shoulders and keep your head up, planting both feet firmly on the floor with your knees slightly apart *(left, 1)*. Avoid slouching, crossing your legs or letting your head, shoulders or upper back slump forward—any of which curve the spine *(left, 2)*. If you must sit for a long period, stand up every once in a while to ease the stress on the back.

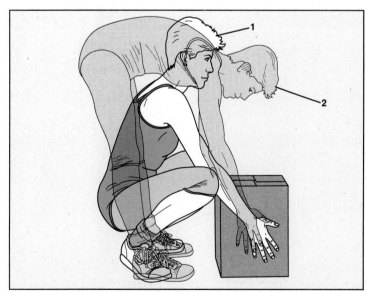

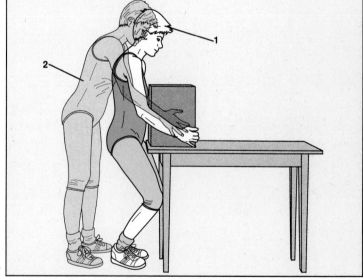

Lifting properly. It is easy to injure the back by lifting an object incorrectly. Whenever you lift an object, position yourself under the weight of it, using your legs rather than your back for leverage. To lift an object off the ground, stand facing it with your feet slightly apart, then squat down and extend your arms to grasp it firmly *(above left, 1)*. With your back straight and your head up, stand straight up, holding the object as close to your body as possible. Never bend down from the waist to pick up an object *(above left, 2)*. To lift an object off a raised surface, stand facing it, then bend your knees slightly, lowering yourself to a level at which you can extend your arms to grasp it firmly *(above right, 1)*. With your back straight and your head up, stand straight up, holding the object as close to your body as possible. Never lean forward from the waist to pick up an object *(above right, 2)*. If you have difficulty lifting any object, stop immediately and find a helper who can assist you.

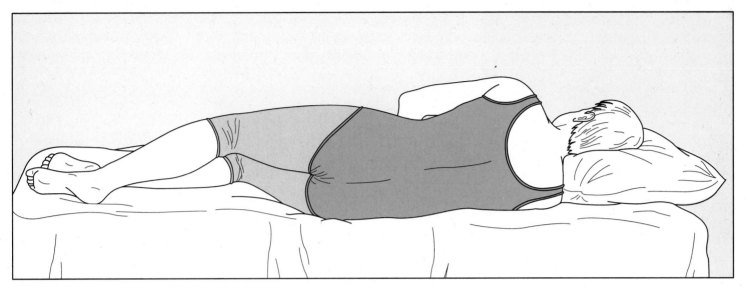

Sleeping properly. Because sleeping is the ultimate form of relaxation for the body, it is easy to forget that improper sleeping posture not only leads to an occasional sore back in the morning, but can create chronic back problems. Ensure that any bed on which you sleep has a firm mattress; if necessary, place a plywood sheet between the mattress and box spring for extra support. Use a firm pillow that is just thick enough to keep your neck and spine aligned when you lie with your head on it; too many pillows or no pillow can misalign the neck and spine, curving the spine. To sleep properly and minimize stress on your back, lie on your side with your knees drawn up slightly *(above)*; if you must sleep on your back, raise your knees slightly and insert a pillow under them. Avoid sleeping on your stomach, especially on a soft mattress; a sway-backed posture can result.

RELIEVING A MUSCLE CRAMP

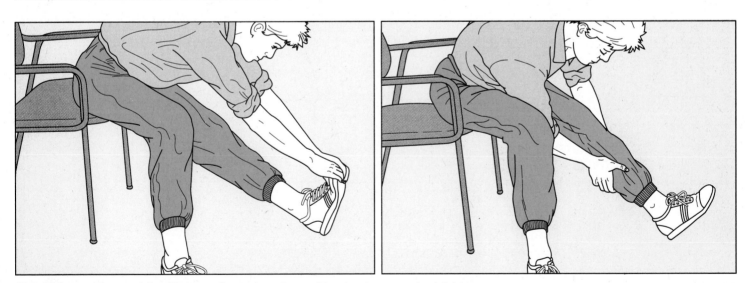

Stretching and massaging the muscle. A cramp is a sudden, involuntary and painful muscle contraction, usually due to chilling or overexertion of the muscle. To relieve a cramp, quickly and gently stretch the muscle in the direction opposite to the contraction. To relieve a cramp in a calf muscle, straighten the leg and gently pull the toes toward the knee *(above, left)*, stretching the muscle. Then, gently massage the muscle thoroughly *(above, right)*. Continue the same way, alternately stretching and massaging the muscle, until the cramp is relieved. To relieve a cramp in a thigh muscle, straighten the leg, then use one hand to pull the toes toward the knee while using the other hand to simultaneously press down on the knee. To relieve a cramp in a foot muscle, straighten the leg and stand up on the foot, then press down firmly on the heel and toe. To relieve any remaining soreness in a muscle after relieving a cramp, apply heat *(page 110)*. Consult a physician about any muscle that is prone to frequent cramps.

RELIEVING MUSCLE TENSION

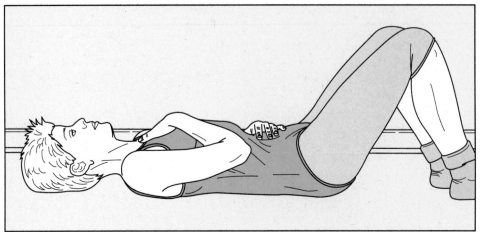

1 **Deep breathing.** Use relaxation exercises to relieve muscle tension. Start with a deep-breathing exercise. Lie on your back and bend your knees, placing your feet flat on the floor 12 inches apart. Resting one hand on your chest and the other hand on your stomach *(left)*, breathe normally for several minutes. Without lifting your shoulders off the floor, begin deep breathing. Inhale slowly to the count of 4, concentrating on the stretch of your chest muscles. Then, exhale slowly to the count of 4, squeezing air out of your lungs by drawing in with your chest and stomach muscles. Repeat the procedure four times, stretching the chest muscles and squeezing air out of the lungs a little more rigorously each time. Breathe normally for several minutes, then sit up slowly.

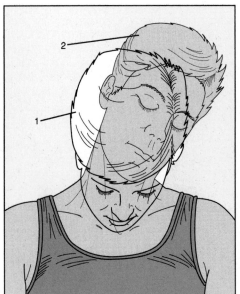 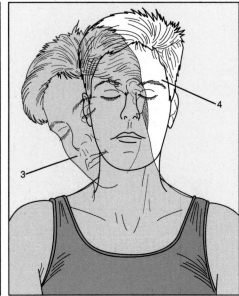

2 **Stretching the neck.** Continue with a neck-stretching exercise. Sitting up straight on a sturdy chair, slowly stretch one side of the neck, then the other. Without moving your back or shoulders, bend your head forward and stop when you feel a stretch in your neck. Hold your head steady *(far left, 1)* to the count of 4. Rotate your head to one side and stop when your ear is directly above the shoulder. Hold your head steady *(far left, 2)* to the count of 4. Rotate your head back to an upright center position, then hold it steady to the count of 4. Follow the same procedure to stretch the other side of the neck, bending your head forward, rotating it to the other side *(near left, 3)* and rotating it back to an upright center position *(near left, 4)*. Repeat the exercise four times.

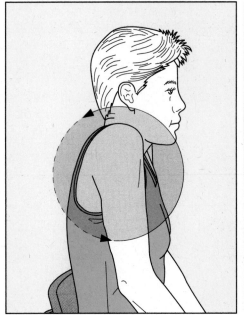 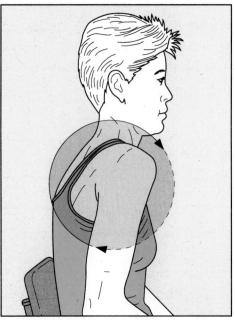

3 **Stretching the shoulders.** Finish with a shoulder-stretching exercise. Sitting up straight on a sturdy chair with your hands on your lap, slowly stretch the shoulders by doing a series of backward rotations, then a series of forward rotations. To do backward rotations *(far left)*, hold your neck and back still. Using a smooth, continuous motion, push the shoulders forward as far as possible, then lift them up, pull them back and drop them down again. Continue the same way to make four complete rotations. To do forward rotations *(near left)*, use the same smooth, continuous motion to pull the shoulders back as far as possible, then to lift them up, push them forward and drop them down again. Continue the same way to make four complete rotations.

PREVENTING A FOOT OR ANKLE PROBLEM

Caring for the feet and ankles. The feet and ankles are the unsung heroes of the musculoskeletal system. The complex network of bones, muscles and ligaments of which the feet and ankles are comprised permits them to support the body's weight and act as shock absorbers for the rest of its skeletal frame. Give the feet and ankles the care they deserve.

Wear proper footwear—and never sacrifice comfort for fashion. Ill-fitting shoes can lead to problems such as bunions, corns, calluses and blisters; in the long term, ill-fitting shoes can cause malformations such as fallen arches. In general, a properly-fitting shoe should: be 1/2 inch longer than the longest toe to keep the tips of the toes from touching the front of the shoe; have a front that is wide enough to permit all the toes to be wiggled freely when standing; have a back that fits snugly around the heel without cutting into it; and provide solid arch support. Avoid wearing a shoe with a heel higher than 2 inches and ensure that any heel is broad enough to stand on without wobbling; a shoe with a high, narrow heel places stress on the ankle and foot, altering the posture in ways that can create back problems.

Clean and groom the feet properly. Wash the feet and wear clean socks or stockings daily; clip the toenails weekly. Pamper tired and sore or swollen feet after any prolonged standing or walking. Soak the feet in a basin of warm—not hot—water and pat them dry with a clean towel. Then, massage the feet using a moisturizing cream to ease muscle tension, and keep the skin soft and supple. Treat any ingrown toenail, corn or callus *(page 100)* and any bunion or heel spur *(page 40)* yourself; consult a physician about any persistent or painful problem.

Ensure that any physical activity in which you engage regularly is not harmful to the feet and ankles, especially if your feet and ankles are weak. Fitness activities such as high-impact aerobics and racket sports, for example, put stress on the feet and ankles without strengthening them. To build strength, exercise the feet and ankles properly *(step below)*.

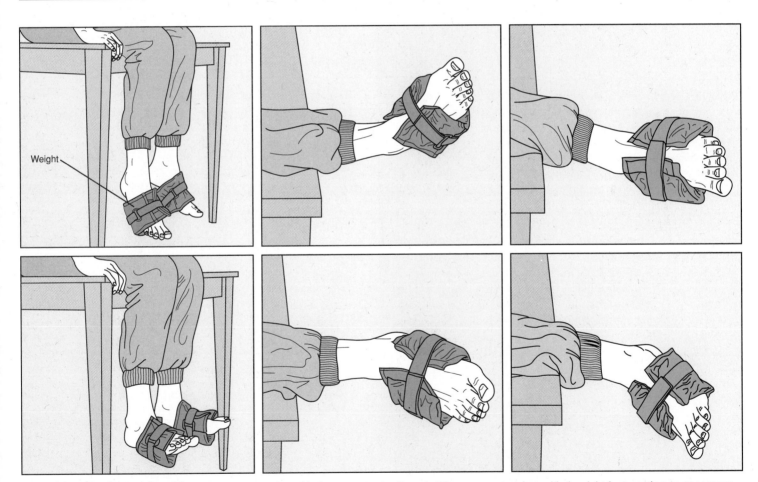

Weight

Exercising the feet and ankles. To build strength and help prevent fatigue or injury, exercise your feet and ankles regularly. Use a pair of 2-pound weights, available at an exercise equipment center. Remove any footwear and attach a weight to each foot, then sit on the edge of a sturdy table that is high enough to keep the feet from touching the floor.

Begin with 50 stretches, resting as necessary. To do a stretch, hold the legs still and pivot the ankles to point the toes down *(left, top)*, then up *(left, bottom)*. To continue, lie stretched out on your right side on the table, your ankles and feet just over the edge of it. Bend the left leg back, then do 50 one-way stretches with the right foot, resting as necessary. To do a one-way stretch, hold the leg still and pivot the ankle to point the toes up *(center, top)*, then relax the ankle to lower the toes to their orginal position *(center, bottom)*. Lying in the same position, bend the right leg back and extend the left leg, then do 50 two-way stretches with the left foot, resting as necessary. To do a two-way stretch, hold the leg still and pivot the ankle to point the toes up *(right, top)*, then down *(right, bottom)*. To finish, lie on your left side to do one-way stretches with the left foot and two-way stretches with the right foot.

NERVOUS SYSTEM

Your nervous system—the brain and the thousands of nerves that connect it to the body—coordinates the complex activities of every part of your body. The diagram on page 49 illustrates the main components of the nervous system. The brain, brain stem and spinal cord form what is called the central nervous system; a network of nerves organized into major nerve groups forms what is called the peripheral nervous system, connecting the central nervous system to the muscles and organs of the body.

Each nerve of the peripheral nervous system is made up of hundreds of different fibers or neurons: sensory neurons that carry messages from a muscle or organ through the spinal cord to the brain; motor neurons that carry messages from the brain back to the muscle or organ. The brain performs the complex function of interpreting these incoming messages, coordinating and transmitting responses, and simultaneously engaging in conscious thought involving memory, learning, thinking and reasoning.

Because the brain is safely encased within the bones of the skull and the nerves are well-protected by a sheath of material called myelin, the nervous system is not easily exposed to the types of irritants and infections that can affect other systems of the body. The list of health tips at right covers basic guidelines to help prevent disorders of the nervous system. In general, a sound body and healthy mental functioning go a long way to preventing the development of a nervous system problem: Avoid stress, eat and sleep well, and exercise regularly.

The Troubleshooting Guide on page 50 puts procedures for minor ailments of the nervous system at your fingertips and refers you to pages 51 to 55 for more detailed information. If headaches, for example, are an occasional problem for you or a family member, familiarize yourself with the steps that can be taken to treat and prevent a headache—whether a migraine or sinus headache *(page 54)* or a tension headache *(page 55)*. Know how to assist an epileptic person during and after a convulsion *(page 52)*. Be alert to the early warning signs of an emotional disorder *(page 51)* and dementia *(page 53)*; consult a physician as soon as possible for a thorough diagnosis of a problem and an appropriate course of treatment for it. For techniques on handling a life-threatening emergency such as a suspected spinal injury, stroke or loss of consciousness, consult the Emergency Guide *(page 8)*. For techniques on caring for a family member who is ill or recuperating from an illness, consult the Equipment & Techniques chapter *(page 110)*.

If you must cope with a disorder of the nervous system at home, do not hesitate to call for help; medical professionals can answer questions concerning symptoms and treatments. Post the telephone numbers for your physician, local hospital emergency room, ambulance and pharmacy near the telephone; in most regions, dial 911 in the event of a life-threatening emergency. For general information about emotional disorders, contact the local chapter of the Mental Health Association in your community.

HEALTH TIPS

1. To help maintain your overall health and a nervous system that functions properly, eat a well-balanced diet.

2. To help you relax and handle stress effectively, get plenty of exercise and fresh air every day—without overdoing it. Walk rather than drive, for example; or, take up a pastime such as swimming, cycling or gardening, choosing an activity to suit your tastes and physical strength.

3. Get plenty of sleep every night. To ensure that you sleep well at night, make the room as dark and quiet as possible; get up at a regular time every morning, avoid taking naps in the afternoon and do not engage in work or other stimulating activity before bedtime.

4. Avoid using nonprescription sleeping pills unless recommended by your physician. If you have trouble sleeping, get up and occupy yourself with a relaxing activity such as reading or taking a warm bath; or, have a light snack such as a glass of milk or a banana.

5. Minimize the use of alcohol and stimulants such as caffeine that act directly on the nervous system.

6. Avoid using a nonprescription medication to treat a chronic fatigue, insomnia or weight problem unless recommended by your physician; some preparations may have adverse effects, especially if used improperly.

7. To prevent mishaps that can damage the brain and nervous system, minimize the chance of a slip or fall by maintaining a safe household. Keep floors and stairs clutter-free. Use no-slip mats and handrails in bathtubs and shower stalls. Work carefully in high places and when using ladders.

8. To prevent serious damage to the brain and nervous system from an accident, always wear a seat belt when riding in a car, a heavy-duty crash helmet when riding on a motorcycle and a light crash helmet when riding on a bicycle.

9. Be aware of any family history of a nervous system problem that can be hereditary—epilepsy, muscular dystrophy, Parkinson's disease or multiple sclerosis, for example. A person at risk should have regular medical examinations to detect early warning signs of any problem.

10. Consult a physician about any potentially-serious symptom of a nervous system problem such as a loss of sensation or movement in a part of the body, recurrent muscular weakness, or loss of muscle coordination or control.

11. Follow the physician's directions to use any prescription medication for a nervous system problem; use the amount specified at the prescribed times and report any side effect to the physician.

12. Never ignore an indication of an emotional or mental disturbance in a family member. If a person shows signs of impaired functioning, do not hesitate to talk to him calmly and confidentially; if necessary, consult a physician as soon as possible to determine the nature of the problem.

NERVOUS SYSTEM

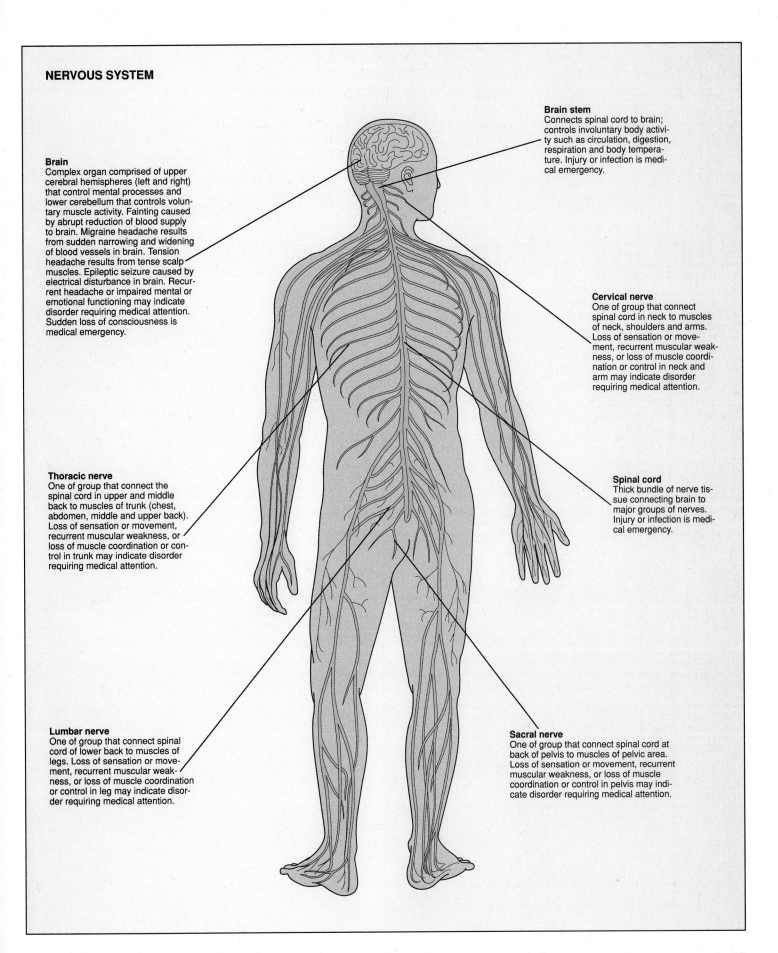

Brain stem
Connects spinal cord to brain; controls involuntary body activity such as circulation, digestion, respiration and body temperature. Injury or infection is medical emergency.

Brain
Complex organ comprised of upper cerebral hemispheres (left and right) that control mental processes and lower cerebellum that controls voluntary muscle activity. Fainting caused by abrupt reduction of blood supply to brain. Migraine headache results from sudden narrowing and widening of blood vessels in brain. Tension headache results from tense scalp muscles. Epileptic seizure caused by electrical disturbance in brain. Recurrent headache or impaired mental or emotional functioning may indicate disorder requiring medical attention. Sudden loss of consciousness is medical emergency.

Cervical nerve
One of group that connect spinal cord in neck to muscles of neck, shoulders and arms. Loss of sensation or movement, recurrent muscular weakness, or loss of muscle coordination or control in neck and arm may indicate disorder requiring medical attention.

Thoracic nerve
One of group that connect the spinal cord in upper and middle back to muscles of trunk (chest, abdomen, middle and upper back). Loss of sensation or movement, recurrent muscular weakness, or loss of muscle coordination or control in trunk may indicate disorder requiring medical attention.

Spinal cord
Thick bundle of nerve tissue connecting brain to major groups of nerves. Injury or infection is medical emergency.

Lumbar nerve
One of group that connect spinal cord of lower back to muscles of legs. Loss of sensation or movement, recurrent muscular weakness, or loss of muscle coordination or control in leg may indicate disorder requiring medical attention.

Sacral nerve
One of group that connect spinal cord at back of pelvis to muscles of pelvic area. Loss of sensation or movement, recurrent muscular weakness, or loss of muscle coordination or control in pelvis may indicate disorder requiring medical attention.

TROUBLESHOOTING GUIDE

PROBLEM	PROCEDURE
Emotional disorder suspected in adult: onset of abnormal behavior	Seek emergency help ✚ if abnormal behavior follows head injury or victim appears violent or capable of injuring self or others
	Monitor emotional patterns *(p. 51)*
	Consult a physician if abnormal behavior severe or becomes chronic
Emotional disorder suspected in child: onset of abnormal behavior	Seek emergency help ✚ if abnormal behavior follows head injury or victim appears violent or capable of injuring self or others
	Consult a physician
Epileptic seizure suspected: sudden staggering, aimless movement or garbled speech and confusion lasting several minutes	Seek emergency help ✚ if seizure follows head injury
	Keep victim resting calmly until disorientation passes and full awareness returns
	Consult a physician if victim not a diagnosed epileptic or seizures of diagnosed epileptic appear to increase in frequency, intensity or duration
Epileptic seizure suspected in child: sudden loss of consciousness and fluttering eyelids lasting 10 to 30 seconds	Keep victim resting calmly until disorientation passes and full awareness returns
	Consult a physician if child not a diagnosed epileptic or seizures of diagnosed epileptic appear to increase in frequency, intensity or duration
Epileptic seizure suspected: sudden loss of consciousness and convulsion lasting several minutes	Seek emergency help ✚ if seizure follows head injury or victim is infant, pregnant or diabetic, or not a diagnosed epileptic
	Treat epileptic seizure *(p. 52)*
	Seek emergency help ✚ if convulsion lasts longer than 5 minutes or victim does not regain consciousness within 5 minutes after convulsion
	Consult a physician if diagnosed epileptic has another seizure within 24 hours or his seizures appear to increase in frequency, intensity or duration
Dementia suspected: gradual onset of forgetfulness and mental confusion; may be accompanied by abnormal behavior	Seek emergency help ✚ if memory loss or confusion follows a head injury
	Consult a physician for thorough diagnosis and appropriate course of treatment
	Manage victim of pre-senile (Alzheimer's disease) or senile dementia *(p. 53)*
Migraine headache suspected: severe, throbbing pain centered inside skull; occurs in morning; preceded by visual disturbance; accompanied by sensitivity to light	Seek emergency help ✚ if headache follows head injury or accompanied by high fever, pain and stiffness of neck or back, or vomiting
	Treat migraine *(p. 54)*
	Watch for and treat any secondary problem
	Consult a physician if headache lasts more than 2 days
Cluster headache suspected: severe, continuous pain centered behind eye; occurs during sleep; accompanied by nasal blockage	Seek emergency help ✚ if headache follows head injury or accompanied by high fever, pain and stiffness of neck or back, or vomiting
	Avoid stress and alcohol; use a nonprescription pain-reliever *(p. 121)*
	Watch for and treat any secondary problem
	Consult a physician if headache lasts more than 2 days
Sinus headache suspected: painful congestion centered in forehead or cheeks, worsened by lowering of head; may occur following common cold or exposure to allergen; accompanied by nasal blockage and discharge	Treat sinus headache *(p. 54)*
	Watch for and treat any secondary problem
	Consult a physician if headache lasts more than 2 days
Tension headache suspected: painful tension across scalp or down back of head and neck; occurs in evening or following period of intense concentration	Treat tension headache *(p. 55)*
	Watch for and treat any secondary problem
	Consult a physician if headache lasts more than 2 days
Neuralgia suspected: severe stabbing pain along length of nerve, especially in side of face, back, buttock or leg	Consult a physician
Paralysis	Seek emergency help ✚
	If necessary, use emergency first aid *(p. 8)*
Loss of consciousness	Seek emergency help ✚
	If necessary, use emergency first aid *(p. 8)*
Speech slurred	Consult a physician

✚ **Medical emergency**

PROBLEM	PROCEDURE
Unexplained loss of muscle control, muscular weakness, numbness or tingling in part of body; movement difficult or uncoordinated	Seek emergency help ✚ if loss of muscle control follows injury
	Consult a physician
Convulsion	Seek emergency help ✚ if convulsion follows head injury or victim is infant, pregnant or diabetic, or not a diagnosed epileptic
	Treat epileptic seizure (p. 52)
	Seek emergency help ✚ if convulsion lasts longer than 5 minutes or victim does not regain consciousness within 5 minutes after convulsion
	Consult a physician if diagnosed epileptic has another seizure within 24 hours or his seizures appear to increase in frequency, intensity or duration
Unexplained drowsiness	Seek emergency help ✚ if drowsiness follows head injury
	Watch for and treat any secondary problem
	Consult a physician if episode severe or recurs
Vision blurred	Seek emergency help ✚ if blurred vision follows head injury
	Watch for and treat any secondary problem
	Consult a physician if episode severe or recurs

✚ Medical emergency

MONITORING EMOTIONAL PATTERNS

Detecting the early warning signs of an emotional disorder. Emotional ups and downs are normal, without lasting consequences for most people. Everyone occasionally suffers from "the blues" or has an emotional outburst. However, because the mental and emotional makeups of individuals differ, not everyone deals with life's exigencies the same way.

For some individuals, a stressful event such as a death, a job loss, retirement, or a severe illness or accident may trigger emotional problems. In other cases, a physical disorder of the brain or nervous system may trigger emotional problems. Adolescents can be particularly prone to emotional disturbances that may be manifested as depression or suicidal tendencies; or, among adolescent females, eating disorders such as anorexia nervosa or bulimia.

Never treat any sign of an emotional disturbance as unimportant. If you feel that someone you love is having difficulty coping with life, discuss it calmly and confidentially. If a problem appears to be persistent or severe, consult a physician as soon as possible. A physician can determine whether an emotional problem is due to a treatable physical disorder or whether it is a mental disorder requiring medication, individual or family therapy, or, in an extreme case, institutionalization. There are self-help and support groups for victims of emotional disorders in most communities; to find one in your area, ask your physician.

Be sensitive to the emotional patterns of your loved ones. Refer to the guidelines below to help you identify the early warning signs of a possible emotional disorder:

• **Depression.** A person becomes unusually apathetic, listless or withdrawn and may be prone to tearfulness. The person may: sleep a lot and at unusual times; lose his appetite; lose interest in sex; or, avoid responsibilities, people and social events.

• **Agitation.** A person becomes unusually anxious, irritable, restless or overactive. The person may have difficulty sleeping or concentrating on work or other responsibilities and be prone to sharp emotional outbursts.

• **Aggression.** A person becomes unusually rebellious or may become unpredictably and abnormally abusive, either verbally or physically. The person may show abnormally flagrant disregard for safety, authority and convention.

• **Delusions.** A person begins to express strong beliefs in what appear to be highly unlikely events—for example, an unrealistically pervasive belief that others are persecuting him (paranoia).

• **Compulsiveness.** A person exhibits a pervasive tendency to engage in what appear to be unnecessarily exaggerated or even irrational habits. The person may attach what appears to be a disproportionate and highly emotional importance to habits such as cleanliness or tidiness, for example.

• **Guilt.** A person expresses unusually extreme feelings of culpability and even self-hatred for what appear to be imagined offenses or inadequacies, especially following a catastrophe or death.

• **Secretiveness.** A person becomes abnormally guarded with other people and may react with suspicion or defensiveness to what appears to others as a harmless question or polite inquiry.

• **Poor self-esteem.** A person expresses unusually strong and exaggerated opinions of his own worthlessness, ineffectiveness, inadequacy or incompetence and seems to have a generalized view of himself as a failure.

TREATING AN EPILEPTIC SEIZURE

Understanding an epileptic seizure. A seizure is an electrical disturbance of the brain that causes sudden, often dramatic motor and psychological changes in a victim, ranging from momentary disorientation to blackouts and convulsions. A seizure can be a temporary reaction to a problem such as a head injury, insulin shock (diabetes), high fever, a brain infection or a drug; recurrent seizures with no treatable cause are called epilepsy. The most severe type of epileptic seizure is a tonic-clonic (grand mal) seizure.

The seizure often begins with the victim experiencing a brief "aura" or warning sensation—typically a sensory hallucination—after which he loses consciousness, falls and convulses for as long as 5 minutes. After the convulsion, the victim remains unconscious for up to 5 more minutes and may remain confused or drowsy for several hours after regaining consciousness. While an epileptic seizure can be a frightening experience, it is usually not a medical emergency and can be managed following the steps below.

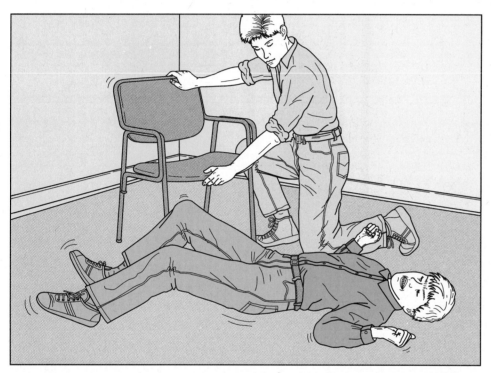

1 **Assisting during a convulsion.** Immediately seek emergency help if a victim is not a diagnosed epileptic or is pregnant, diabetic or injured. To prevent injury to a victim when he loses consciousness, catch him as he is about to fall, if possible, then immediately and gently lay him down. While the victim convulses, quickly clear away any nearby movable objects *(left)*; if necessary, quickly shift him away from any dangerous immovable object such as a wall, stairway or piece of heavy furniture or equipment. During the convulsion—which may last 5 minutes—stand aside and interfere as little as possible; if the victim vomits, immediately turn him on his side to prevent choking. Do not try to hold the victim down; do not try to pry open his jaw to force anything between his teeth—even if he appears to be biting his tongue. Immediately seek emergency help if the convulsion lasts more than 5 minutes; otherwise, assist the victim when the convulsion ends *(step 2)*.

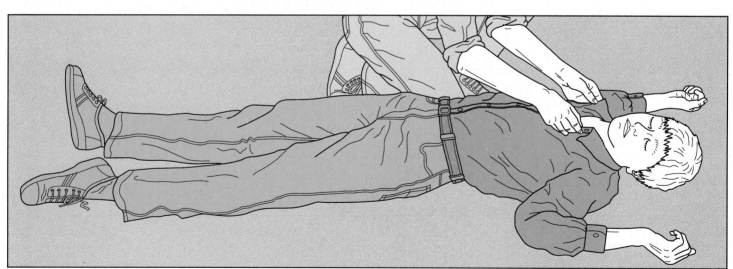

2 **Assisting after a convulsion.** When the convulsion ends, stay nearby and let the victim sleep until he regains consciousness—this may take 5 minutes. Loosen the victim's clothing at the neck *(above)*, chest and waist, then place him in the recovery position *(page 22)*. Immediately seek emergency help if the victim has another convulsion before regaining consciousness or does not regain consciousness after 5 minutes. Otherwise, once the victim is conscious, keep him resting calmly until any disorientation has passed and he is fully aware of his surroundings. If necessary, clean up any urine or vomit, and stop the bleeding from any minor injury sustained during the convulsion. Consult a physician if there is another seizure within 24 hours or if the frequency of seizures appears to be increasing.

MONITORING AND TREATING DEMENTIA

Managing dementia. Most people suffer an occasional memory lapse, but a person who exhibits increasing memory deterioration, mental confusion and odd behavior is said to be suffering from dementia—which occurs when brain cells begin to die in large numbers. Deterioration of the brain is a normal result of aging (senile dementia); it may also occur in younger adults (pre-senile dementia) due to a disorder such as a tumor or Alzheimer's dis-ease. The early stages of dementia are characterized by subtle behavior changes that may go unnoticed by family members; it is often an outsider who notices the changes—increasing forgetfulness about recent events; confusion about times and places; heightened irritability or suspiciousness; and declining initiative or interest in everyday activities. To help you manage a suspected condition of dementia, refer to the guidelines below:

• **Diagnosing dementia.** If you notice signs of possible dementia in a family member, consult a physician; if the dementia is due to a treatable disorder that is diagnosed early, it may be stoppable and even reversible. If the dementia is due to a disorder such as Alzheimer's disease and is not reversible, family members will need to take steps to begin managing the disorder.

• **Managing early stages of dementia.** With family support, a victim of mild dementia can lead a relatively normal home life. Become as well-informed as possible about any disorder such as Alzheimer's disease that is causing the dementia; ask your physician about a support group in your community. Take steps to assist the victim *(step below, left)*, as much as possible minimizing the effects of forgetfulness and confusion on daily routines. Ensure that the victim follows the physician's directions to use any medication for the symptoms of the dementia and reports any side effect to the physician.

• **Managing later stages of dementia.** As dementia progresses, a victim's behavior may become unpredictable. Sudden tears, depressions and paranoia are common. The victim's thinking may become disorganized and delusionary. Communication with the victim may become increasingly difficult. The victim may have difficulty with tasks such as dressing, eating and hygiene. Family members may need to supervise the victim daily and take steps to protect him *(step below, right)*. It may be necessary to have community service-providers help with meals, cleaning or shopping.

• **Managing advanced dementia.** With advanced dementia, a victim may be physically and mentally disabled. The victim may be unable to speak, understand or recognize people or places. There may be increasing immobility, loss of muscle control and incontinence. Like a child, the victim may require constant care and supervision. Continuous nursing care may be needed. If the victim is immobilized, physiotherapy may need to be arranged.

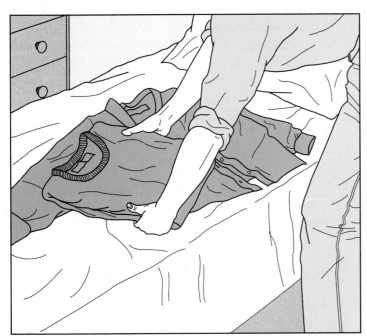

Assisting a victim during the early stages. In the early stages of dementia, take steps to ease the forgetfulness and confusion that may keep the victim from performing daily tasks. To combat forgetfulness, for example, make lists of things to be done, mark events to be remembered on a calendar, write out instructions and give gentle verbal reminders. Keep daily routines as consistent as possible. Encourage the victim to keep up with recreational activities and hobbies; if former activities are too difficult, help the victim find substitutes—minimally a daily walk. Assist with personal grooming by helping the victim choose appropriate clothing *(above)*, for example, or by placing a brush, toothbrush or razor in a place where it will be seen and used.

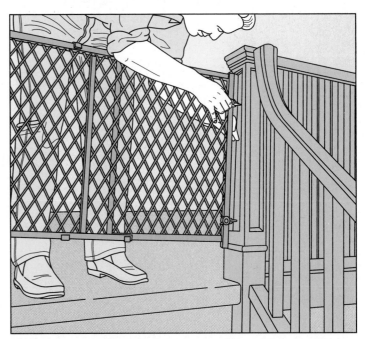

Protecting a victim during the later stages. In the later stages of dementia, take steps to prevent the victim from injuring himself due to mental confusion and physical carelessness. For example, barricade a stairway *(above)* to prevent a fall. Keep sharp knives or potentially dangerous utensils and tools out of reach. Keep poisons and medications locked away. To minimize the risk of fire, help the victim who smokes to stop smoking; never let him smoke unsupervised. To eliminate the possibility of scalds, lower the thermostat on the hot water heater and supervise the victim's use of any heating or cooking appliance. Sew address labels on the inside of the victim's clothing in the event that he wanders off and becomes lost.

TREATING MIGRAINE

Managing a migraine condition. Migraine is a type of recurrent and often severe headache that can last several hours to several days. The symptoms of migraine may include a "premonition" of the attack—typically a visual disturbance such as flashing lights or zigzag lines—followed by a momentary numbness or tingling of one side of the head or body; then, the onset of a severe, throbbing headache that may be accompanied by sensitivity to light, nausea and dizziness.

• To help relieve a migraine attack, lie down in a dark room and rest completely; if necessary, use a nonprescription pain-reliever *(page 121)*. During a prolonged attack, eat only small, light meals; if you are worried, do not hesitate to consult a physician.

• Try to identify any trigger for a migraine attack. Keep a diary of daily sleeping, eating and working patterns, noting events such as weather changes, emotional stresses and rigorous physical activities; isolate factors that may contribute to the onset of a migraine. Jot down the time and suspected cause of an attack as well as the nature of the symptoms for discussion with a physician.

• Talk to your physician about tests to ensure that no other physical disorder is the cause of migraine attacks. Ask the physician to check your blood pressure to ensure that high blood pressure is not the cause; he may also decide to do blood tests or X-rays.

• Cut your intake of food that may trigger migraine attacks. In general, avoid cheese, chocolate, alcohol and citrus fruits unless you are sure that they do not trigger your migraines.

The initial symptoms of migraine are produced by a sudden narrowing of the blood vessels of the brain; the migraine headache itself occurs when the blood vessels widen again and begin to throb as the blood flow is restored, putting pressure on the surrounding brain tissue. While there is no medical cure for migraine, the frequency and severity of an attack can be minimized. To help you or a family member manage a migraine condition, refer to the guidelines below:

• To prevent the onset of a migraine attack, minimize stress and lead as routine a life as possible. Maintain proper, regular sleeping and eating habits, and exercise regularly.

• If you are prescribed a prescription medication for your migraine condition, carefully follow the physician's directions to use only the amount specified at exactly the prescribed times. Some medications are to be taken only when a migraine attack begins, while other medications are to be taken regularly to prevent a migraine attack from developing.

• Closely monitor the effects of any prescription medication for your migraine condition. Note any side effects or any change in how quickly or well the medication relieves a symptom and report the information to the physician—a different form, dosage or type of medication may be necessary to treat your migraine condition.

• If you are worried that migraine attacks are beginning to seriously disrupt your daily life, join a support group for migraine sufferers; to find a support group in your community, ask your physician.

TREATING A SINUS HEADACHE

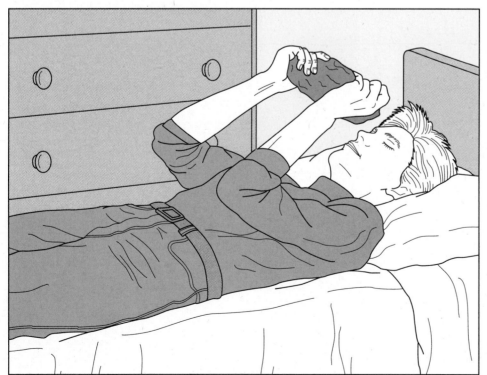

Relieving sinusitis. Sinusitis causes a persistent pain in the forehead or cheeks that is made worse by stooping, lying down or coughing and that may be accompanied by a stuffy, runny nose. Consult a physician if the pain is severe. Otherwise, relieve the sinusitis for 48 hours to try and clear it up. Stop any smoking *(page 70)* and minimize exposure to dust and other airborne irritants. Get plenty of rest. If necessary, use a nonprescription pain-reliever *(page 121)*. To provide spot-relief from blocked sinuses and stuffy nasal passages, use a hot compress. Soak a clean facecloth in hot—not scalding—water and wring it out, then fold it into a pad. Lean back in a comfortable chair or lie down, then position the compress *(left)* to cover the forehead, eyes and cheekbones, leaving it in place for 10 minutes. Reheat the compress and repeat the application as often as necessary. Consult a physician if any pain or a fever *(page 114)* persists for more than 48 hours.

TREATING A TENSION HEADACHE

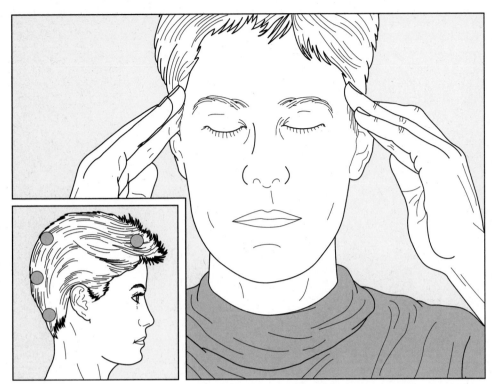

1 Massaging the scalp. A tension headache causes a sensation of tension and aching or pain that extends from the forehead back across the scalp or across the scalp down the back of the head. To relieve a tension headache, minimize any stress by resting; take a warm bath or lie down in a dark room. If necessary, use a nonprescription pain-reliever *(page 121)*. For additional relief, do a series of gentle massages to relax the muscles. Starting with a scalp massage, sit upright in a chair and close your eyes. Placing your fingertips on your temples *(left)*, gently massage them using a slow, circular motion. Working back around the ears in an arc to the base of the skull, massage the scalp at points every few inches the same way. Reposition your fingertips just above your temples and repeat the procedure, massaging the scalp at points along a parallel arc slightly higher than the first one. Continue the same way, repositioning your fingertips slightly higher above your temples each time and making sure you massage each of the main pressure points of the scalp *(inset)*.

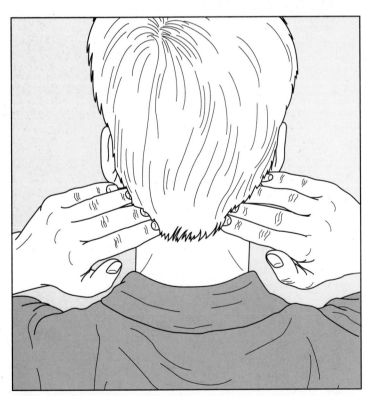

2 Massaging the neck. After massaging the scalp, continue by massaging the neck. Take a deep breath and release it fully, relaxing your chest and shoulders; take several more breaths and release them the same way. Tilt the head back slightly to relax the neck muscles. Placing your fingertips just beneath the base of the skull on each side of the spine *(above)*, gently massage the neck using a slow, circular motion. Working down the neck in a line to the base of it, massage at points every few inches the same way. Repeat the massage, using slightly greater pressure than the first time.

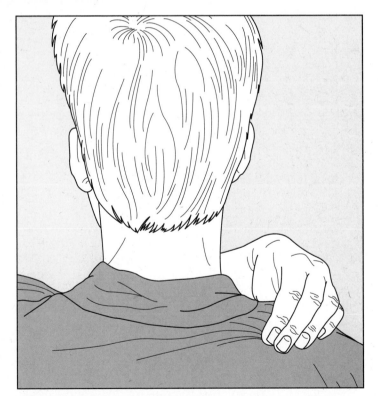

3 Massaging the shoulders. After massaging the neck, continue by massaging the shoulders one at a time. To massage a shoulder, relax the arm, laying the hand in your lap. Using the opposite hand, work from the outer edge of the shoulder to the base of the neck, gently kneading the shoulder muscle. Use a pinching motion to massage the front and back of the muscle simultaneously *(above)*, then a circular motion to massage the top of it. Repeat the massage, using slightly greater pressure than the first time. Massage the other shoulder following the same procedure.

CIRCULATORY SYSTEM

Your circulatory system consists of your heart and the thousands of miles of arteries, veins and capillaries that carry blood to every part of your body. Blood flowing through the lungs absorbs oxygen, then returns to the heart and is pumped via the aorta through a network of arteries to the tiny capillaries at every extremity of the body. The capillaries pass oxygen from the blood to body tissue and pick up waste carbon dioxide. The blood is then carried by a network of veins back to the heart, where it is pumped back to the lungs to give up carbon dioxide and pick up oxygen. The lymphatic system is a network of channels alongside the circulatory system that contain a fluid called lymph; the lymph carries different types of cells that are used to attack infectious disease organisms that enter the body. Refer to the diagrams of the circulatory and lymphatic systems on page 57.

Circulatory and lymphatic system disorders are not everyday medical problems for the average household. Every family, however, should take steps to prevent the development of disorders that can affect either system. The list of health tips at right covers basic guidelines for preventing circulatory diseases and minimizing the risk of infectious diseases that put strain on the lymphatic system. Take steps to guard against the development of heart disease *(page 59)* and hypertension *(page 60)* among family members. Ensure that family members are vaccinated against infectious diseases *(page 63)*; be alert to the early warning signs of a possible infectious disease *(page 62)*.

The Troubleshooting Guide on page 58 puts procedures for minor circulatory disorders and infectious diseases at your fingertips and refers you to pages 59 to 63 for more detailed information. Familiarize yourself with the procedures for treating a fainting spell *(page 59)* or, if requested by your physician, for self-monitoring blood pressure *(page 60)*. Consult a physician for a diagnosis of any suspected infectious disease; properly treat any common infectious disease at home yourself *(page 63)*. For techniques on handling a life-threatening emergency such as a heart attack, stroke or shock, consult the Emergency Guide *(page 8)*. For techniques on caring for a family member recuperating from an illness, consult the Equipment & Techniques chapter *(page 110)*.

If you must cope with a circulatory disorder or infectious disease in the home, do not hesitate to call for help; medical professionals can answer questions concerning symptoms and treatments. Post the telephone numbers for your physician, local hospital emergency room, ambulance and pharmacy near the telephone; in most regions, dial 911 in the event of a life-threatening emergency. For general information on circulatory disorders, contact a local chapter of the American Heart Association in your community.

SAFETY TIPS

1. To prevent the development of heart disease, stop any smoking *(page 70)*. Smoking is one of the leading causes of heart and respiratory disease.

2. Hypertension—or chronic high blood pressure—is a risk factor for the development of heart and kidney disease and stroke. To help detect and treat a hypertension problem before it becomes serious, have your blood pressure checked at least once each year; twice each year after the age of 50.

3. To maintain overall health and prevent heart problems, eat a well-balanced diet, cutting down on foods that contain saturated fats—fats that remain solid at room temperature.

4. Prevent the development of hypertension and heart disease by maintaining your body weight within an acceptable range *(page 35)*; excess body weight places extra demands on the circulatory system.

5. To help prevent a circulatory problem such as hypertension, reduce your consumption of salt; for example, substitute lemon juice, pepper or other spices for table salt. Eat fresh food, substituting it for processed food; when you choose processed food, read the label carefully and avoid using types with high salt content.

6. The American Heart Association recommends moderate exercise as a way of preventing hypertension. Get plenty of fresh air and exercise every day—without overdoing it. Walk rather than drive, for example, or choose a relaxing activity to suit your personal tastes and physical strength.

7. To enhance overall fitness and reduce the chances of developing hypertension or heart disease, minimize the amount of stress in your life by using relaxation techniques.

8. Prevent the development of an infectious disease of the digestive tract *(page 72)* due to food contamination by handling food properly. Do not share eating implements, drinking glasses, towels or cosmetics. Wash the hands well with soap and water after using the bathroom and before eating.

9. To prevent the development of an infectious disease, properly treat any skin wound *(page 100)*. Wash the wound thoroughly with soap and water, then bandage it. Consult a physician about the need for possible tetanus treatment if the wound is caused by a dirty or rusty object; about the need for possible rabies treatment if the wound is caused by an animal.

10. Prevent the development of infectious disease from sexual activity with proper genital and sexual hygiene; use a condom to reduce the risk of contracting a disease *(page 84)*.

11. To prevent the development of infectious diseases, ensure that you and your family members are properly immunized throughout infancy, childhood and adulthood *(page 63)*.

12. Carefully follow the physician's directions to use any prescription medication for a circulatory system problem or an infectious disease; use the amount specified at the prescribed times and report any side effect to the physician.

CIRCULATORY SYSTEM

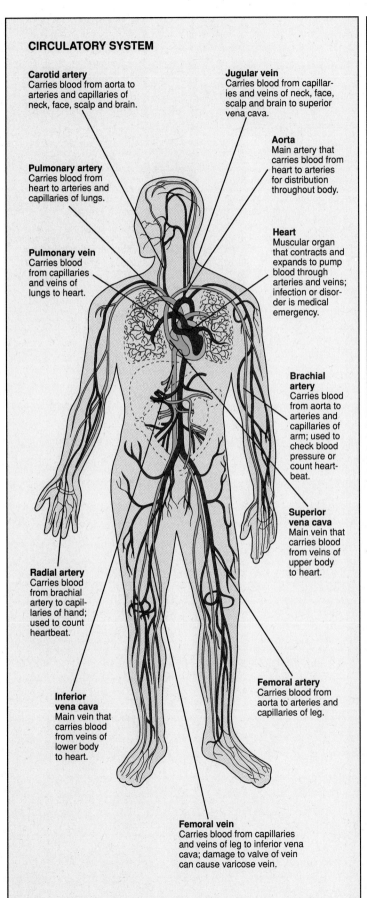

Carotid artery
Carries blood from aorta to arteries and capillaries of neck, face, scalp and brain.

Pulmonary artery
Carries blood from heart to arteries and capillaries of lungs.

Pulmonary vein
Carries blood from capillaries and veins of lungs to heart.

Radial artery
Carries blood from brachial artery to capillaries of hand; used to count heartbeat.

Inferior vena cava
Main vein that carries blood from veins of lower body to heart.

Jugular vein
Carries blood from capillaries and veins of neck, face, scalp and brain to superior vena cava.

Aorta
Main artery that carries blood from heart to arteries for distribution throughout body.

Heart
Muscular organ that contracts and expands to pump blood through arteries and veins; infection or disorder is medical emergency.

Brachial artery
Carries blood from aorta to arteries and capillaries of arm; used to check blood pressure or count heartbeat.

Superior vena cava
Main vein that carries blood from veins of upper body to heart.

Femoral artery
Carries blood from aorta to arteries and capillaries of leg.

Femoral vein
Carries blood from capillaries and veins of leg to inferior vena cava; damage to valve of vein can cause varicose vein.

LYMPHATIC SYSTEM

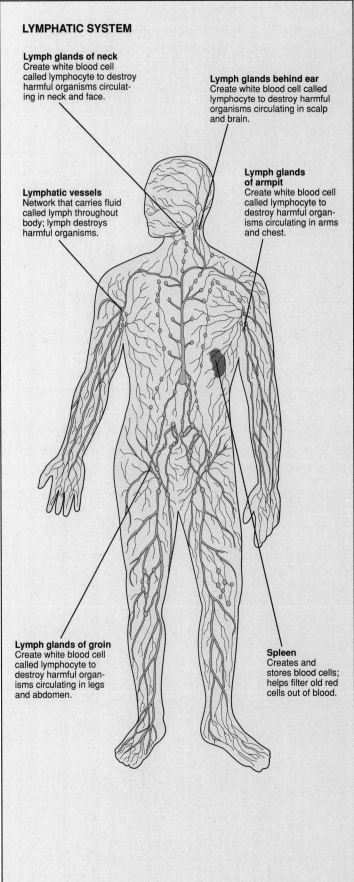

Lymph glands of neck
Create white blood cell called lymphocyte to destroy harmful organisms circulating in neck and face.

Lymphatic vessels
Network that carries fluid called lymph throughout body; lymph destroys harmful organisms.

Lymph glands behind ear
Create white blood cell called lymphocyte to destroy harmful organisms circulating in scalp and brain.

Lymph glands of armpit
Create white blood cell called lymphocyte to destroy harmful organisms circulating in arms and chest.

Lymph glands of groin
Create white blood cell called lymphocyte to destroy harmful organisms circulating in legs and abdomen.

Spleen
Creates and stores blood cells; helps filter old red cells out of blood.

TROUBLESHOOTING GUIDE

PROBLEM	PROCEDURE
Family history of heart disease	Prevent heart disease (p. 59) and hypertension (p. 60)
Family history of hypertension	Prevent hypertension (p. 60)
Fainting spell suspected: pallor; sweaty, cold or clammy skin; shallow or uneven breathing; dizziness; numbness or tingling	Treat fainting spell (p. 59)
	Consult a physician if fainting spell unexplained or recurs
Heart attack suspected: tightness or pain across chest; labored breathing; weak or irregular pulse; cold or clammy skin	Seek emergency help ✚
	If necessary, use emergency first aid (p. 8)
Heart rhythm unusual or uncomfortable	Consult a physician; prevent heart disease (p. 59)
Chest pain	Consult a physician; prevent heart disease (p. 59)
Breath shortness	Consult a physician; prevent heart disease (p. 59)
Sweating heavy; unexplained	Consult a physician; prevent heart disease (p. 59)
Stroke suspected: disorientation; paralysis or weakness on one side of body; speaking, swallowing or breathing difficulty	Seek emergency help ✚
	If necessary, use emergency first aid (p. 8)
Shock suspected: trauma; injury; illness; sudden emotional upset	Seek emergency help ✚
	If necessary, use emergency first aid (p. 8)
Profuse bleeding: spurting, bright red blood or gushing, burgundy blood	Seek emergency help ✚
	If necessary, use emergency first aid (p. 8)
Loss of appetite	Rest; drink fluids
	Watch for any infectious disease (p. 62)
	Consult a physician if appetite loss of child for more than 1 day; of adult for more than 1 week
Listlessness or fatigue	Rest; drink fluids
	Watch for any infectious disease (p. 62)
	Consult a physician if listlessness or fatigue lasts more than 1 week
Muscle or joint achiness	Rest; drink fluids
	Watch for any infectious disease (p. 62)
	Consult a physician if achiness lasts more than 1 week
Rash	Consult a physician
Mumps suspected: painful and swollen salivary gland at front of ear, under jaw or under tongue	Consult a physician
	Treat mumps (p. 63)
	Prevent infectious diseases (p. 63)
Chickenpox suspected: itchy rash of pink, raised spots that blister and scab; starts on trunk and spreads to arms, legs and head	Consult a physician
	Treat chickenpox (p. 63)
	Prevent infectious diseases (p. 63)
Rubella (German measles) suspected: rash of pink, raised spots; starts behind ears and spreads to rest of body	Consult a physician
	Treat rubella (p. 63)
	Prevent infectious diseases (p. 63)
Measles suspected: white spots inside cheeks, then rash of pink, raised spots; starts behind ears and spreads to rest of body	Consult a physician
	Treat measles (p. 63)
	Prevent infectious diseases (p. 63)
Influenza suspected: achiness, fever and sweating, then chest congestion, coughing and sneezing	Consult a physician
	Treat influenza (p. 63)
	Prevent infectious diseases (p. 63)
Infectious mononucleosis suspected: lethargy, achiness, loss of appetite and fever, then persistent sore throat	Consult a physician
	Treat infectious mononucleosis (p. 63)

✚ Medical emergency

PREVENTING HEART DISEASE

Minimizing risks of heart disease. Although the heart is one of the strongest muscles of the body, like any other muscle it can be weakened and damaged by improper treatment. Recent medical research indicates that lifestyle choices can have significant effects on long-term coronary health. Smoking, for example, as well as excessive consumption of alcohol, caffeine, salt, sugar or fat, can contribute to the development of heart disease. Other studies indicate that particular groups of people are at high risk for the development of heart disease: those with Type A personalities—highly driven, competitive and time-conscious; those with a family history of heart attack or stroke in the 30- to 50-year age bracket; women after menopause; and, those 65 years and older. Heart disease among children and adolescents is much rarer than among older adults and is usually due to congenital, or birth-related, heart defects, or is rheumatic in nature—occurring as a delayed reaction to serious illness. Any adult 40 years of age or older, especially one at risk for the development of heart disease, should take steps to monitor his health and adjust his lifestyle in order to prevent the development of disease. Information on the proper prevention of heart disease is readily available from your physician or the American Heart Association. Refer to the guidelines below to help you take the steps necessary to prevent the development of a heart disorder:

● **Minimizing health risks.** A healthy lifestyle is the best long-term guarantee against the development of heart disease. In particular, teach children the importance of healthy habits that can provide the basis for a long and healthy adult life. Eat a well-balanced diet, maintaining your weight within the recommended range *(page 35)*. Avoid excessive use of alcohol *(page 35)*. Stop any smoking *(page 70)*. Get plenty of fresh air and exercise, without overdoing it; choose a physical activity that suits your taste and capacity *(page 32)*. Get regular and adequate amounts of sleep and relaxation, and minimize stress *(page 33)*.

● **Having regular checkups.** Any adult 40 years of age or older should request a thorough heart examination as a part of an annual medical checkup. The physician will listen to your heart using a stethoscope to detect any abnormality; he may also send you for an electrocardiogram to get more detailed information about your heart. Ensure that the physician checks your blood pressure and informs you of the result; if the blood pressure is elevated, ask about follow-up appointments to be examined for possible hypertension *(page 60)*.

● **Learning the warning signs.** Be aware of and alert to the physical symptoms that may indicate the development of heart disease. Consult a physician as soon as possible about any of the following: a marked or uncomfortable change in heart rhythm; intermittent pain in the chest, particularly if it tends to radiate to the neck, the jaw, a shoulder or an arm; recurrent shortness of breath, particularly if it tends to occur while at rest or after only slight exertion; recurrent and unexplained dizziness or fainting spells; or, recurrent episodes of unexplained, heavy sweating.

TREATING A FAINTING SPELL

Handling fainting spells. A fainting spell is a self-correcting form of mild shock that occurs when the blood supply to the brain drops, resulting in partial or complete loss of consciousness. A range of conditions can provoke a fainting spell—including overheating, fatigue, hunger or sudden emotional upset.

Although a fainting spell is seldom serious, the victim can sustain an injury if he loses consciousness without notice. Often, the victim may exhibit signs of an impending fainting spell just prior to it; if detected, action can be taken quickly *(step right)* and he may not lose consciousness. Signs of an impending fainting spell include:

● Extreme pallor

● Sweating—beads of perspiration

● Cold or clammy skin

● Shallow or uneven breathing

● Dizziness or lightheadedness

● Numbness or tingling of the hands or feet

● Nausea

● Visual disturbances—images dark or blurry

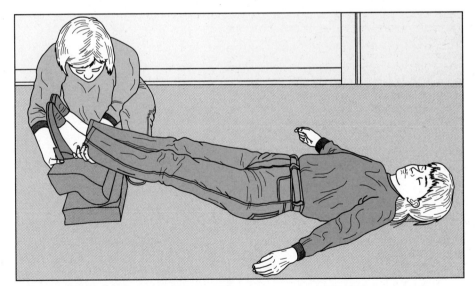

Assisting the victim of a fainting spell. If the victim exhibits signs of an impending fainting spell, take him to a well-ventilated area—outdoors, if possible. Have the victim lie down on his back with his legs elevated, resting his feet on books *(above)* or pillows. Loosen the victim's clothing at the neck, chest and waist. If the victim suffers a fainting spell, monitor his vital life signs *(page 12)*, checking for breathing and taking a pulse; keep others away. Apply a cool cloth to the victim's face. If the victim does not recover within 2 minutes, seek emergency help. When the victim is conscious, give him sips of water and keep him resting calmly until any disorientation has passed and he is fully aware of his surroundings. Consult a physician about a fainting spell with no obvious cause or recurring fainting spells.

PREVENTING HYPERTENSION

Minimizing the risk of hypertension. An estimated 35 million Americans suffer from hypertension—chronic high blood pressure. Because hypertension tends to have no symptoms until the blood pressure is extremely high, when it can cause dizziness and headaches, many individuals remain unaware of their condition. Without treatment, however, hypertension can eventually lead to the development of heart disease, stroke and kidney disease.

• **Minimizing health risks.** A healthy lifestyle is the best guarantee against the development of hypertension. Eat a well-balanced diet low in salt and maintain your recommended weight *(page 35)*. Avoid excessive use of alcohol *(page 35)*. Stop any smoking *(page 70)*. Get plenty of exercise, without overdoing it; choose an activity that suits your taste and capacity *(page 32)*. Get an adequate amount of rest and minimize stress *(page 33)*.

• **Monitoring blood pressure.** If you are between 30 and 50 years of age, have your blood pressure measured once a year; if you are more than 50 years of age, have it measured twice annually. Ask the physician to tell you the result. If your blood pressure is elevated, schedule a follow-up appointment to check whether it is chronically elevated; the physician may want to take measurements of your blood pressure over a period of time and may request that you self-monitor it *(step below)* to facilitate a diagnosis.

Persons most at risk for the development of hypertension typically have a family history of hypertension. Other factors related to the development of hypertension include obesity, excess alcohol consumption, smoking, use of the contraceptive pill and stress. If you are 30 years of age or older, you should take steps to prevent the development of hypertension—especially if you are at high risk. Refer to the information presented below:

• **Treating hypertension.** If a physician diagnoses you as having hypertension, he will usually perform additional tests to determine whether there is another physical disorder causing it, then treat the physical disorder to help eliminate the hypertension. However, in the vast majority of cases of hypertension, there is no identifiable cause and the typical method of control will usually include the following: regular medical appointments to check the blood pressure; self-monitoring of the blood pressure between medical appointments; dietary changes such as a reduction in salt and alcohol intake; stress-reduction techniques; and prescription medication. To successfully control a diagnosed condition of hypertension, carefully follow the physician's directions to use any prescription medication for it; always use only the amount specified at only the prescribed times, reporting any side effect to the physician. If you are required to self-monitor your blood pressure at home, ensure that you follow the proper procedures *(step below)*.

SELF-MONITORING BLOOD PRESSURE

Monitoring the blood pressure at home.
If you are required to self-monitor your blood pressure to help your physician diagnose or treat a condition of hypertension, use the recommended blood pressure monitoring device: an electronic-display type *(step 2)* or a pressure-gauge type *(step 3)*. Ask the physician to demonstrate the proper use of the device recommended, carefully following the manufacturer's directions for it; have the physician observe and correct your technique until it is right, if necessary.

Prior to measuring your blood pressure *(step right)*, ensure that you take the steps necessary to do the reading properly:

• Do not smoke, eat, drink or exercise within 15 minutes of measuring your blood pressure.

• Measure your blood pressure in a cool, quiet location when you feel relaxed.

• Always measure your blood pressure using the same arm—whichever arm is most comfortable for you to use.

• Measure the blood pressure at the times specified by the physician and always at the same times; take a series of 2 to 3 readings each time at intervals of 2 minutes.

• Keep a careful record of your blood pressure measurements, including the date and time of each series of readings.

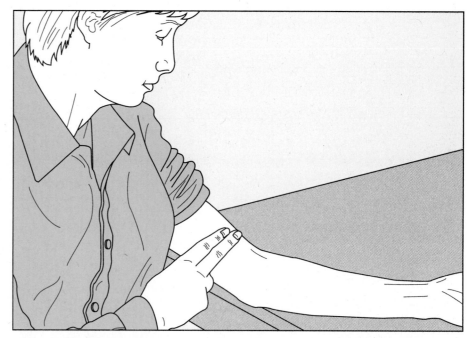

1 Locating the brachial artery. To prepare for measuring your blood pressure, remove the clothing from your upper arm, pushing up the sleeve or taking off your shirt. Sit with the arm bent and resting on a table, then locate the brachial artery. Making a fist with the hand of the arm, use the index and middle fingers of the other hand to feel for the artery; lightly press the fingertips against points on the inside of the upper arm about 1 inch above the crease of the elbow *(above)*, noting the point at which you feel the pulse of the artery. Then, take your blood pressure reading at the point using your electronic-display type *(step 2)* or pressure-gauge type *(step 3)* blood-pressure monitoring device.

SELF-MONITORING BLOOD PRESSURE (continued)

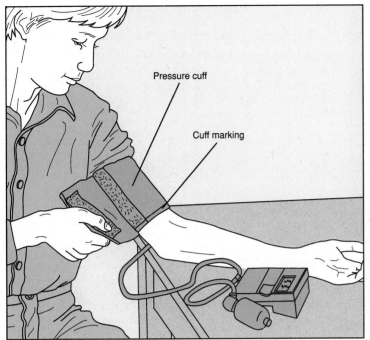

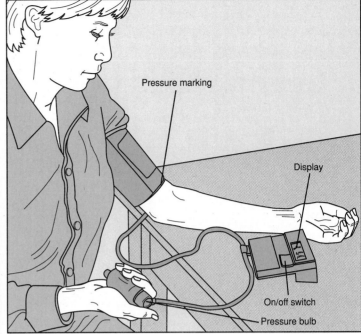

2 **Taking a reading with an electronic-display device.** With the arm bent and resting on the table at heart level, wrap the cuff of your device snugly around the upper arm 2 inches above the crease of the elbow *(above, left)*; for the device shown, ensure that the cuff marking lies against the brachial artery *(step 1)*. Switch on the display unit, then use your free hand to squeeze-pump the pressure bulb to fill the cuff, stopping when the number 170 appears in the display unit window. Release the pressure bulb to decrease the cuff pressure *(above, right)*; the device will automatically calculate your blood pressure and display it as two numbers in the window. The larger number is the systolic pressure when the heart contracts; the smaller number is the diastolic pressure when the heart relaxes. The blood pressure is the ratio of the systolic pressure to the diastolic pressure. If the numbers 120 and 80 appear, for example, your blood pressure is 120/80.

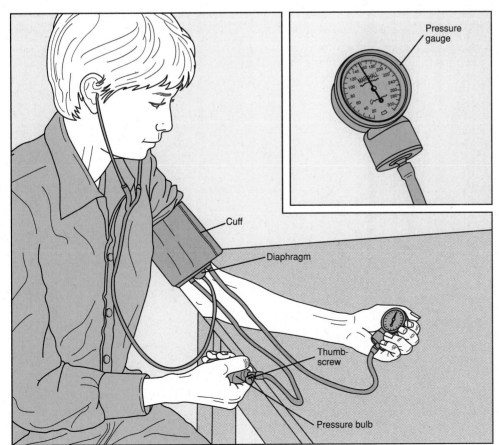

3 **Taking a reading with a pressure-gauge device.** With the arm bent and resting on the table at heart level, wrap the cuff of your device snugly around the upper arm 2 inches above the crease of the elbow, then hold the pressure gauge lightly with the hand. Put on the stethescope and fit its diaphragm under the cuff against the brachial artery *(step 1)*. Holding the pressure bulb in your free hand, tighten the thumbscrew, then squeeze-pump the pressure bulb to fill the cuff *(left)*; stop when the pressure gauge needle *(inset)* reaches the 170 position. To measure your blood pressure, loosen the thumbscrew just enough to let the pressure gauge needle slowly swing back toward 0. Listening carefully with the stethescope, note the numerical position of the needle when you hear the first beat of the pulse—the systolic pressure when the heart contracts. Continue listening to the pulse, noting the numerical position of the needle when you hear the last beat of the pulse—the diastolic pressure when the heart relaxes. The blood pressure is the ratio of the systolic pressure to the diastolic pressure. For example, if you hear the first beat when the needle indicates 120 and the last beat when it indicates 80, your blood pressure is 120/80.

RECOGNIZING INFECTIOUS DISEASES

Recognizing the warning signs of an infectious disease.
Harmful foreign organisms such as bacteria, viruses, fungi and parasites abound in the environment and can gain entry to the body in many ways. Foreign organisms are breathed into the respiratory system; they enter the digestive system with the foods we eat and by means of activities such as kissing. Foreign organisms on the skin can enter the body through an open wound; an insect such as a mosquito that punctures the skin can also inject harmful organisms. The reproductive system can be exposed to foreign organisms through sexual contact.

Whether an organism that enters the body causes illness depends on its degree of toxicity or virulence and on the capacity of the immune system to defend the body against it. An inability to defend the body against an infectious organism means that a person develops full-blown symptoms of disease, usually after an incubation period. These symptoms may be quite varied: vomiting or diarrhea for an infection of the digestive system; congestion, coughing or sneezing for a respiratory infection; an inflammation or rash for a skin infection.

Prior to the onset of full-blown symptoms of an infectious disease, a person during the incubation period may exhibit early warning signs of infection—low-level symptoms that typically precede the development of most infectious diseases. To help prevent the spread of an infectious disease, be alert to the early warning signs listed below, reducing the person's level of activity and contact with others as soon as they are detected:

- Loss of appetite

- Listlessness, fatigue or irritability

- Headache

- Aching muscles or joints

- Fever *(page 114)*

- Swollen lymph glands *(step below)*

CHECKING THE LYMPH GLANDS

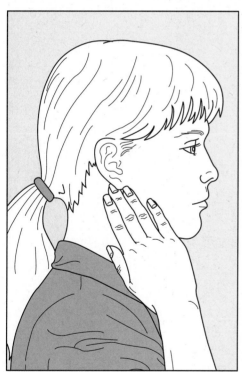 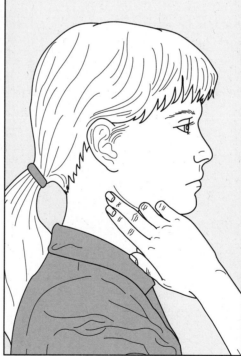 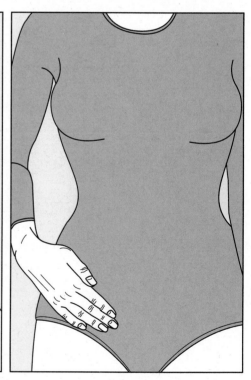

Checking for swollen lymph glands. Lymph glands are located throughout the body; they are responsible for collecting and breaking down bacteria, viruses, dust and other noxious substances circulating in the blood that are picked up from the respiratory system, the digestive system and the skin. When a lymph gland is working to destroy many foreign organisms at the same time—such as at the onset of an infectious disease—it may become swollen and tender or painful. If you suspect that a person is becoming ill, you should check the lymph glands for signs of swelling. Place the tips of the fingers against the lymph gland behind the base of the ear *(above, left)*, below the back of the jaw *(above, center)* and in the joint of the groin between the leg and abdomen *(above, right)*. Press in firmly against each lymph gland, using a circular motion to palpate it. Check the lymph gland under the arm in the center of the armpit the same way. Consult a physician if any lymph gland is swollen, tender or painful.

PREVENTING INFECTIOUS DISEASES

Vaccinating against infectious diseases. To minimize the risk of contracting a dangerous infectious disease, a person should be properly vaccinated through infancy and childhood; an adult needs a vaccination booster against diphtheria and tetanus every 10 years after adolescence. Use the checklist at right to help assess the vaccination status of family members. Vaccinations are also recommended for an adult against Hepatitis B; annually for a person over the age of 65 against influenza; for a person traveling abroad against any infectious disease endemic to a region he visits.

Consult a physician to arrange for a vaccination. A vaccination typically takes only minutes, with the physician usually injecting the vaccine; an exception is polio vaccine, administered orally. Have the physician record the type and dose of vaccine administered as well as the vaccination date on an official state vaccination record form; use the form to record any future vaccinations the same way. Ask the physician about expected side effects of the vaccination such as a fever or rash, or soreness at the site of an injection. Call the physician immediately if any side effect is severe or persists.

AGE	VACCINATION
2 months	Diphtheria-tetanus-pertussis, first dose; polio, first dose
4 months	Diphtheria-tetanus-pertussis, second dose; polio, second dose
6 months	Diphtheria-tetanus-pertussis, third dose
12 months	Tuberculosis test; if necessary, vaccination
15 months	Measles-mumps-rubella
18 months	Diphtheria-tetanus-pertussis, fourth dose; polio, third dose; hemophilus influenza B
4 to 6 years (pre-school)	Diphtheria-tetanus-pertussis, fifth dose; polio, fourth dose
10 years	Measles-mumps-rubella, booster if never infected with measles
14 to 16 years, then once every 10 years	Diphtheria-tetanus, booster

TREATING INFECTIOUS DISEASES

Managing common infectious diseases. Every household must deal with an occasional infectious disease in a family member. Children, in particular, are prone to infections due to their still-developing immunity and frequent exposure to infectious agents in daycare or school. Be alert to the early warning signs of an infectious disease *(page 62)*, then consult a physician for a diagnosis.

• **Mumps.** The swelling associated with mumps subsides within 1 week of its onset, but the saliva of an infected person remains infectious to others for 2 weeks longer. Until the swelling subsides, have the person rest and drink fluids. Monitor temperature *(page 114)* and relieve pain or reduce fever by using a nonprescription pain-reliever *(page 121)*. While the person is infectious, avoid any oral contact. Consult a physician about any severe headache, earache, abdominal pain or neck stiffness.

• **Chickenpox.** An infected person remains infectious to others until the entire rash forms scabs, usually within 5 days of its onset; the scabs slowly heal over the next 2 weeks. While the person is infectious, have him rest in bed and drink plenty of fluids. Monitor temperature *(page 114)* and reduce any fever by using a nonprescription pain-reliever *(page 121)*. To relieve itching, apply calamine lotion to the rash; avoid scratching it. Consult a physician if the rash becomes inflamed or pus-filled.

• **Rubella (German measles).** The rash associated with rubella subsides within 5 days of its onset, but an infected person remains infectious to others for 4 days longer. While the person is infectious, have him rest and avoid contact with any pregnant woman. Monitor temperature *(page 114)* and reduce fever by using a nonprescription pain-reliever *(page 121)*. Consult a physician about any severe headache or joint pain.

Prevent contact between an infected person and an infant, pregnant woman or elderly person. Carefully follow the instructions to use any prescription medication to treat an infectious disease; use only the prescribed amount at only the specified times and report any side effect to the physician. Use the guidelines below to help you treat an infectious disease at home:

• **Measles.** An infected person is no longer infectious to others when the rash associated with measles subsides—typically within 1 week of its onset. Until the rash subsides, have the person rest and drink plenty of fluids. Monitor temperature *(page 114)* and reduce fever by using a nonprescription pain-reliever *(page 121)*. Consult a physician about any severe headache or joint pain.

• **Influenza.** The acute symptoms of influenza usually subside within 1 week of their onset, but full recovery may take 1 week longer. Until the symptoms subside, have the person rest and drink plenty of fluids. Monitor temperature *(page 114)* and reduce fever by using a nonprescription pain-reliever *(page 121)*. Relieve any congestion *(page 67)* and cough *(page 69)*. Consult a physician about any severe cough or labored, painful breathing.

• **Infectious mononucleosis.** The acute symptoms of infectious mononucleosis typically subside within 3 weeks of their onset, but full recovery may take 6 weeks or longer. Until the symptoms subside, have the person rest and drink plenty of fluids. Relieve any sore throat *(page 68)*. Monitor temperature *(page 114)* and reduce fever by using a nonprescription pain-reliever *(page 121)*. Until full recovery, avoid oral contact and keep an infected person from rupturing his enlarged spleen by preventing strenuous activity. Consult a physician about a severe sore throat that lasts more than 5 days or any severe headache or neck stiffness.

RESPIRATORY SYSTEM

Your respiratory system consists of the body organs that facilitate breathing—the complex and life-sustaining process by which your body takes oxygen, one of its basic fuels, from the air around you. The diagram on page 65 illustrates the major organs involved in the process. Air inhaled through the nose passes through a nasal cavity and enters the pharynx; air inhaled through the mouth passes over the tongue directly to the pharynx. The air then moves down through a branch-like system of passages into the bronchioles of each lung. At the tips of the bronchioles, tiny, sponge-like sacs conduct a complex exchange, taking oxygen out of the air in the lungs and passing it into the blood, and taking carbon dioxide out of the blood and passing it back into the air in the lungs. As the lungs contract, the waste air is pushed back up to be exhaled.

Because the respiratory system is an easy access route into the body for dust, fumes and microscopic organisms, its organs are prone to infections and ailments of many types. While some respiratory system infections such as the common cold are usually not serious, no respiratory system infection should ever be ignored. Any ailment affects the ability of the respiratory system to provide the body with the oxygen it needs; with improper treatment, an ailment can worsen and lead to secondary complications, especially in an infant or elderly person.

The Troubleshooting Guide *(page 66)* puts procedures for common respiratory ailments at your fingertips and refers you to pages 66 to 71 for more detailed information. Familiarize yourself with the procedures for treating a common cold *(page 66)*. Know how to stop a nosebleed *(page 69)*, how to evaluate and relieve a sore throat *(page 68)*, how to assist an asthmatic person during an asthma attack *(page 69)* and how to deal with a respiratory allergy *(page 71)*. For techniques on handling a life-threatening respiratory emergency such as choking or arrested breathing, consult the Emergency Guide *(page 8)*. For basic techniques on caring for a family member who is ill or recuperating from an illness, consult the Equipment & Techniques chapter *(page 110)*.

The list of health tips at right covers basic guidelines in helping to prevent respiratory ailments and keep the respiratory system in good condition. Smoking, for example, can be virtually the sole cause of many chronic and deadly respiratory problems. If you are a smoker, stop smoking *(page 70)* and give the delicate organs of your respiratory system a chance at dealing effectively with the myriad infectious agents and airborne pollutants from which it protects your body.

If you must cope with a respiratory ailment in the home, do not hesitate to call for help; medical professionals can answer questions concerning symptoms and treatments. Post the telephone numbers for your physician, local hospital emergency room, ambulance and pharmacy near the telephone; in most regions, dial 911 in the event of a life-threatening emergency. Keep handy the telephone number of an ear, nose and throat specialist recommended by your physician. For general information on respiratory ailments, contact a local chapter of the American Lung Association.

HEALTH TIPS

1. To maintain your overall health and help you prevent an infection of your respiratory system, eat and sleep properly, and avoid stress and excessive use of alcohol.

2. To maintain a healthy respiratory system, do not smoke. If you smoke, make every effort to stop *(page 70)*; if necessary, consult a physician about ways to overcome your habit.

3. To strengthen the respiratory system, get plenty of exercise and fresh air—without overdoing it. Walk rather than drive, for example; or, take up a pastime such as gardening, choosing an activity to suit your tastes and physical strength.

4. To prevent respiratory problems, wear respiratory protection *(page 70)* to do dusty work in the house or to use chemicals that emit hazardous vapors.

5. To prevent respiratory problems, minimize daily exposure to dust and airborne irritants. Vacuum and dust the house, and clean furnace, air conditioner and humidifier filters regularly; if you live in a dusty area, install an air-filtration system.

6. Never suppress a sneeze or cough—they are reflexes that expel dust and bacteria from the respiratory system. Never sneeze with your mouth closed.

7. Breathe through your nose, not your mouth; the nasal cavities are designed to warm and moisten incoming air, and filter out dust and bacteria, minimizing stress on the lungs.

8. In general, consult a physician about any respiratory ailment in an infant, a young child or an elderly person.

9. Consult a physician about a respiratory problem accompanied by a potentially–serious symptom such as: recurrent or persistent cough or sore throat; persistent high fever; swollen neck glands; or, painful, difficult breathing.

10. Minimize the spread of a contagious respiratory infection such as a common cold by: using facial tissues instead of handkerchiefs; covering your nose and mouth to sneeze or cough; washing your hands after contact with an infected person, and washing dishes and linens used by the person.

11. Unless recommended by your physician, avoid using a nonprescription medication to treat a common cold; the medication may have negative side effects.

12. Follow the physician's directions to use any prescription medication; use the amount specified at the prescribed times and report any side effect to the physician.

13. If you suffer from a respiratory ailment such as asthma and use a prescription medication, carry a Medic Alert card or wear a Medic Alert bracelet that will allow a medical professional to identify your condition in an emergency.

14. If you suffer from a major respiratory ailment, consult a physician before undertaking a rigorous physical activity; if recommended, consult a physiotherapist about an exercise program to gradually increase your respiratory capacity.

RESPIRATORY SYSTEM

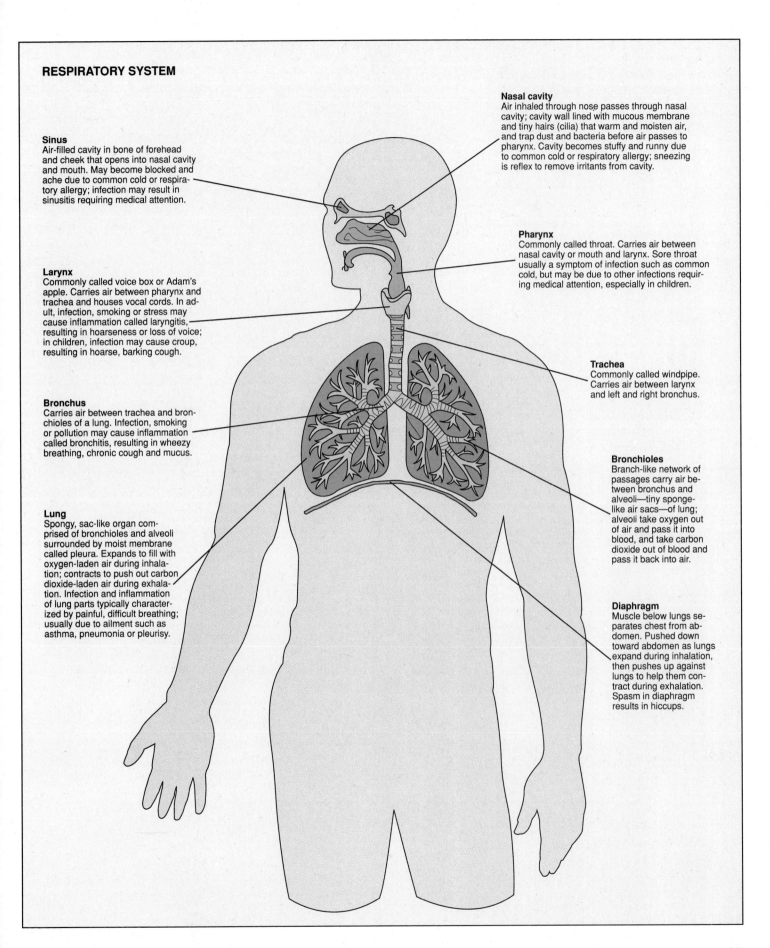

Sinus
Air-filled cavity in bone of forehead and cheek that opens into nasal cavity and mouth. May become blocked and ache due to common cold or respiratory allergy; infection may result in sinusitis requiring medical attention.

Larynx
Commonly called voice box or Adam's apple. Carries air between pharynx and trachea and houses vocal cords. In adult, infection, smoking or stress may cause inflammation called laryngitis, resulting in hoarseness or loss of voice; in children, infection may cause croup, resulting in hoarse, barking cough.

Bronchus
Carries air between trachea and bronchioles of a lung. Infection, smoking or pollution may cause inflammation called bronchitis, resulting in wheezy breathing, chronic cough and mucus.

Lung
Spongy, sac-like organ comprised of bronchioles and alveoli surrounded by moist membrane called pleura. Expands to fill with oxygen-laden air during inhalation; contracts to push out carbon dioxide-laden air during exhalation. Infection and inflammation of lung parts typically characterized by painful, difficult breathing; usually due to ailment such as asthma, pneumonia or pleurisy.

Nasal cavity
Air inhaled through nose passes through nasal cavity; cavity wall lined with mucous membrane and tiny hairs (cilia) that warm and moisten air, and trap dust and bacteria before air passes to pharynx. Cavity becomes stuffy and runny due to common cold or respiratory allergy; sneezing is reflex to remove irritants from cavity.

Pharynx
Commonly called throat. Carries air between nasal cavity or mouth and larynx. Sore throat usually a symptom of infection such as common cold, but may be due to other infections requiring medical attention, especially in children.

Trachea
Commonly called windpipe. Carries air between larynx and left and right bronchus.

Bronchioles
Branch-like network of passages carry air between bronchus and alveoli—tiny sponge-like air sacs—of lung; alveoli take oxygen out of air and pass it into blood, and take carbon dioxide out of blood and pass it back into air.

Diaphragm
Muscle below lungs separates chest from abdomen. Pushed down toward abdomen as lungs expand during inhalation, then pushes up against lungs to help them contract during exhalation. Spasm in diaphragm results in hiccups.

TROUBLESHOOTING GUIDE

PROBLEM	PROCEDURE
Common cold suspected	Monitor and relieve common cold symptoms (p. 66); consult a physician if no improvement in common cold symptoms within 1 week
Laryngitis suspected: hoarse, squeaky or lost voice	Rest, drink plenty of fluids, stop any smoking (p. 70) and avoid using voice
	Consult a physician if hoarse, squeaky or lost voice lasts more than 4 days
Cough with mucus	Monitor and relieve cough (p. 68)
	Consult a physician if mucus bloody, brown or frothy, or cough lasts more than 1 week
Dry cough	Stop any smoking (p. 70)
	Consult a physician if cough lasts more than 1 week
Sore throat	Monitor and relieve sore throat (p. 68)
	Consult a physician if sore throat lasts more than 2 days
Asthma attack suspected: severe, sudden onset of wheezy breathing	Treat asthma attack (p. 69); seek emergency help ✚ if it lasts more than 30 minutes
	Consult a physician to identify and treat possible allergy (p. 71) or infection
Allergic reaction suspected: sneezing; runny, stuffy nose; itchy, watery, swollen eyes; itchy skin rash; wheezy breathing	For severe, wheezy breathing, treat asthma attack (p. 69); seek emergency help ✚ if it lasts more than 30 minutes
	Consult a physician to identify and treat allergy (p. 71)
Breathing difficult: wheezing	If severe, treat asthma attack (p. 69); seek emergency help ✚ if it lasts more than 30 minutes
	Consult a physician to identify and treat possible allergy (p. 71) or infection
Breathing difficult: pain; breathlessness	If severe, seek emergency help ✚; if necessary, use emergency first aid (p. 8)
	Consult a physician to identify and treat infection
Nosebleed	Stop nosebleed (p. 69)
	Consult a physician if nosebleeds frequent

✚ **Medical emergency**

TREATING A COMMON COLD

Monitoring and relieving cold symptoms. The common cold is caused by any one of many different viruses that affect the upper respiratory tract—the nose, sinuses and throat. Because you can contract a cold virus through direct contact with a person who has a cold or by inhaling an airborne virus, your risk of contracting a virus is higher if you are regularly exposed to crowded living and working conditions. Whether you develop a cold after contracting a virus depends on whether you are immune to the particular cold virus to which you have been exposed, as well as on your physical condition; if you are stressed, overtired, eat poorly, smoke or have a chronic illness, your chance of developing a cold is greater. Common cold symptoms include: sneezing; stuffy, runny nose; aching, stuffy head; sore throat; cough; fatigue; loss of appetite; and low-grade fever. Once you develop a common cold, there is no "cure" for it—no medication will eliminate the virus or shorten the duration of the cold. In general, take steps to prevent spreading the virus: Avoid direct contact with other people and wash your hands frequently, especially after blowing your nose; avoid handling food that others will eat. Follow the guidelines below to monitor the progress of a common cold and treat its symptoms:

• Get plenty of rest.

• Drink plenty of fluids, especially water and fruit juices; cut back on the intake of milk products which can thicken secretions of mucus and increase congestion.

• If you smoke, reduce stress on the respiratory system by stopping smoking (page 70).

• Check the neck glands (page 56) and consult a physician if the neck glands are swollen.

• Monitor temperature (page 114) and consult a physician if a fever persists for more than a few days, rises above 101° Fahrenheit or is accompanied by chills.

• Relieve aches and reduce fever by using a nonprescription pain-reliever (page 121) and consult a physician if there is persistent or severe pain in the teeth, sinuses or ear.

• Relieve congestion by using a humidifier and saline nose drops; for an infant, also a nasal aspirator (page 67).

• Monitor and relieve any sore throat (page 68).

• Monitor and relieve any cough (page 69) and consult a physician if coughing is uncontrolled or excessive, or is accompanied by difficult, painful breathing.

• Consult a physician if there is no improvement in symptoms after 7 days or if any symptom remains after 14 days.

RELIEVING CONGESTION

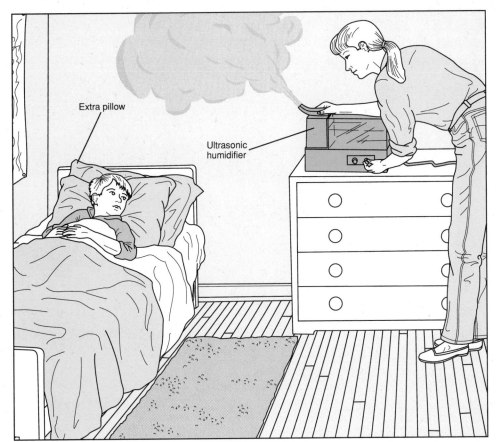

Using a humidifier. To help relieve the congestion of a common cold, use a humidifier such as the ultrasonic type shown; extra humidity can help loosen mucous secretions and clear blocked sinuses, stuffy nasal passages and congested breathing. Use the humidifier wherever a person with a cold rests or sleeps, ensuring you clean it daily *(page 71)*. Following the manufacturer's instructions, set up the humidifier on a steady surface near the person, adjusting any nozzle on it *(left)* to direct a steady flow of mist into the air around the person. **Caution:** Never position a humidifier where a child can grab or tip it. To provide additional relief from congestion during rest or sleep, use an extra pillow to elevate the head slightly.

To provide spot-relief from blocked sinuses and stuffy nasal passages, use a hot compress. Soak a clean facecloth in hot—not scalding—water and wring it out, then fold it into a pad and wrap it with a towel. Hold the compress gently against one side of the nose to cover the cheek and eye, leaving it in place for 10 minutes. Reheat the compress and do the same on the other side of the nose.

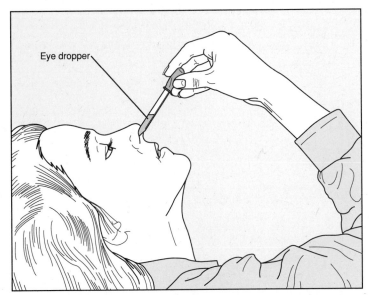

Using saline nose drops. To help relieve the nasal congestion of a common cold, use a fresh solution of saline nose drops in each nostril twice a day. Fill a clean eye dropper with a cool saline solution of 1 teaspoon of salt per cup of boiling water. Tilting the head back as far as possible, insert the tip of the eye dropper into a nostril *(above)* and squeeze 3 drops of the solution into it. Without tilting the head forward, do the same for the other nostril. Keep the head tilted back for 2 to 3 minutes before tilting it forward again. Alternatively, buy nonprescription saline nose drops at a pharmacy and follow the manufacturer's instructions to use them.

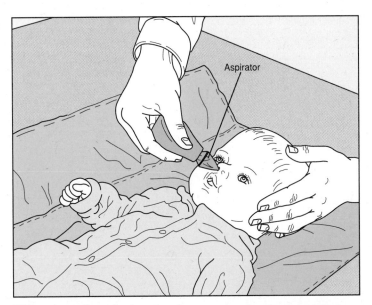

Using a nasal aspirator. To relieve nasal congestion in an infant, lay him on his back; if necessary, have a helper hold the infant's hands to prevent fidgeting. Administer saline nose drops *(step left)*, then clear each nostril twice using a nasal aspirator. To use the aspirator, squeeze its bulb, then gently insert its nozzle into the tip of a nostril *(above)*. **Caution:** Never insert the nozzle without first squeezing the bulb. To extract mucus from the nostril, slowly release the bulb. To drain the aspirator, squeeze the bulb to expel the mucus into a facial tissue, then use a fresh tissue to wipe the nozzle clean. After using the aspirator, wash and rinse it well.

TREATING A SORE THROAT

Monitoring a sore throat. A sore throat due to a common cold is rarely serious unless it persists for more than 4 days; relieve any pain by gargling *(step right)*. However, a sore throat not due to a common cold that is severe or persists for more than 2 days, especially in a child or young adult, may be evidence of a serious infection—tonsillitis, strep throat (streptococcus bacteria) or infectious mononucleosis (Epstein-Barr virus), for example. Monitor a person with a sore throat for symptoms that indicate the need to consult a physician:

• Monitor temperature *(page 114)*; consult a physician if a fever persists for more than 2 days or rises above 101° Fahrenheit.

• Check the neck glands *(page 56)*; consult a physician if they are swollen.

• Inspect the tongue and throat using a tongue depressor and flashlight; consult a physician if they are badly inflamed or have a filmy coating.

• Consult a physician if a sore throat is associated with malaise, fatigue or lethargy.

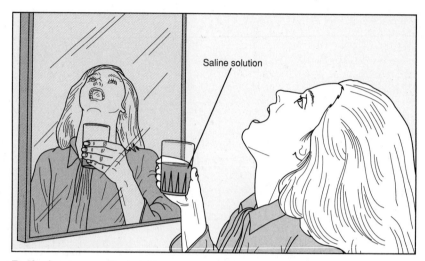

Saline solution

Relieving a sore throat. To temporarily relieve the ache, dryness and tenderness of a sore throat, stop any smoking *(page 70)* and gargle with a fresh mixture of a warm saline solution as often as necessary. Mix a solution of 1 teaspoon of salt per cup of boiling water in a clean glass, then let it cool just enough for it to be sipped without burning the lips or tongue. Stand at a sink to take a mouthful of the solution; without swallowing it, tilt your head back as far as possible. Open your mouth to hold the solution in the back of your throat and gargle vigorously for several seconds *(above)*. Lean forward to spit out the solution. Continue the same way, gargling one mouthful of the solution after another, until the glass is empty. After gargling, wash the glass in hot, soapy water and rinse it well.

TREATING A COUGH

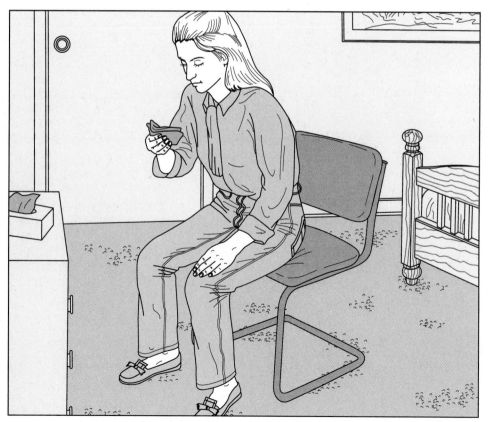

Monitoring and relieving a cough.
A cough that accompanies a common cold is usually not cause for concern; it is a reflex that helps to rid the respiratory tract of mucus and should subside when the mucus is expelled. However, you should seek medical help if any cough: persists for more than 1 week; produces bloody, pink, brown or frothy mucus; is painful or is accompanied by painful or labored breathing; or is accompanied by a persistent fever that rises above 101° Fahrenheit *(page 114)*. Otherwise, avoid using any nonprescription cough suppressant and learn to "cough effectively" to help a cough do its job. Stop any smoking *(page 70)*. Drink plenty of fluids and use a humidifier *(page 67)* to help loosen mucus. Each time you feel a cough coming on, sit on a sturdy chair with both feet firmly on the ground and lean forward slightly *(left)*. Inhale deeply, hold your breath for 5 seconds, and cough twice sharply to expel as much mucus as possible into a clean facial tissue. If a constant cough prevents sleep and leaves you tired or breathless, consult a physician about using medication to relieve it.

TREATING AN ASTHMA ATTACK

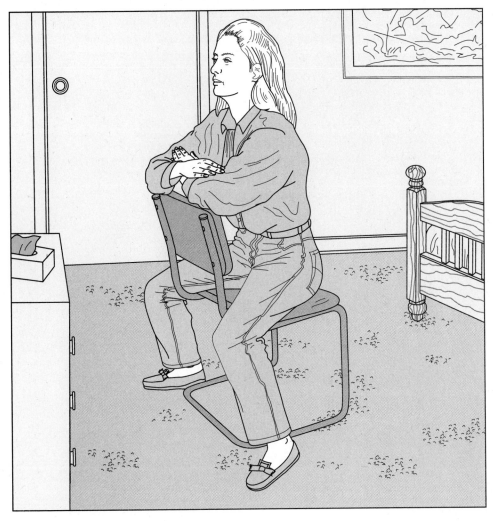

Assisting an asthmatic person. A diagnosed asthmatic under a physician's care uses prescription medication that is usually administered using an inhaler. If an asthmatic has an attack of wheezing and difficulty breathing, assist the person. Stay calm, and keep people and pets away. If necessary, help the person locate and administer any asthma medication, following instructions on the prescription label. To help ease breathing, leave the person to sit straddling a sturdy straight-backed chair, facing the back of it with the arms crossed and resting on the back of it *(left)*—straightening the posture and steadying the ribcage. If possible, open a window or exterior door to increase the supply of fresh air. If the attack lasts longer than 30 minutes, seek medical help.

After an attack, keep the person calm and help identify any "trigger" of the attack—for example, exposure to a possible allergen such as dust, smoke, fumes, pet hair, food or a drug, physical stress due to vigorous exercise, an infection or cold air, or emotional stress. Advise the person to note the time of the attack and any suspected trigger of it for discussion with a physician.

STOPPING A NOSEBLEED

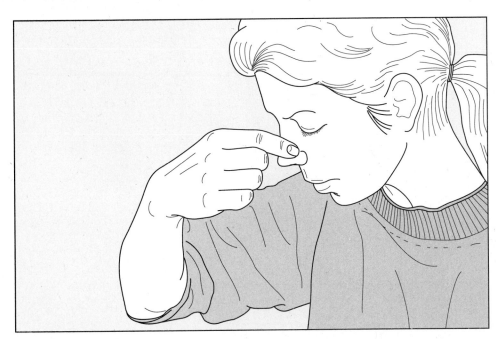

Using pressure to stop a nosebleed. If a nosebleed follows a head injury, use any emergency first aid necessary *(page 8)*. To stop a common nosebleed not due to an injury, have the person sit upright and lean slightly forward. To stop the bleeding, pinch the nostrils just below the bone in the nose *(left)* and breathe through the mouth, spitting out any blood that trickles from the nose into the back of the throat; the bleeding should stop in 5 to 10 minutes. If the bleeding persists, wrap ice cubes in a towel or facecloth and press it gently over the bridge of the nose. If the bleeding still persists, seek medical help. After the bleeding stops, sit quietly for 15 minutes; do not blow the nose for at least 2 hours. If nosebleeds recur frequently, consult a physician.

PREVENTING RESPIRATORY PROBLEMS

Stopping smoking. Most health experts agree that smoking tobacco is one of the most dangerous personal behaviors in which anyone can engage. Three key ingredients of tobacco smoke—tar, nicotine and carbon monoxide—are known causes of major respiratory diseases such as bronchitis, emphysema and lung cancer, and are risk factors for the development of bladder cancer, heart disease and some circulatory disorders. There is also evidence that the "second-hand smoke" produced by smokers is harmful to others who must breathe it, especially infants and children who do not have mature immune systems.

• Make a list of the positive reasons to stop smoking and read it several times a day.

• Analyze your reasons for smoking. Jot down the time, what you are doing, and the way you feel each time you light a cigarette.

• Call your physician and enlist his help. He may prescribe a nicotine-based chewing gum to help you through any withdrawal.

• Get lots of exercise and fresh air.

• Engage in fulfilling activities that make smoking difficult—gardening, for example, or an active sport.

• Use substitution techniques—instead of smoking after eating, brush your teeth.

To prevent the development of major illness and avoid the social stigma attached to being a smoker, consider stopping any smoking habit. There are commercial devices readily available at any pharmacy to help a person stop smoking, and many employers now offer counseling and group programs to help a person break the smoking habit. As well, there are smoking-cessation support groups in most communities; to find one in your area, contact a local chapter of the American Lung Association, the American Heart Association or the American Cancer Society, or ask your physician. Refer to the tips below on stopping smoking:

• Spend time in places that do not allow smoking.

• Use relaxation techniques when you crave a cigarette—take a long, deep breath and hold it for 10 seconds, then exhale slowly.

• Reduce your consumption of coffee, alcohol and other substances that you associate with smoking.

• Satisfy any oral craving by eating vegetables such as carrots or celery, or by chewing gum.

• Each time you resist smoking a cigarette, reward yourself with something you like—but not a cigarette.

• Do not be afraid of failure; if you fail to stop smoking once, keep trying. Every little bit of time that you do not smoke helps.

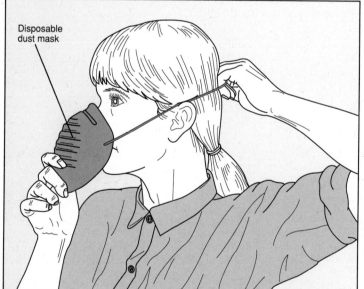

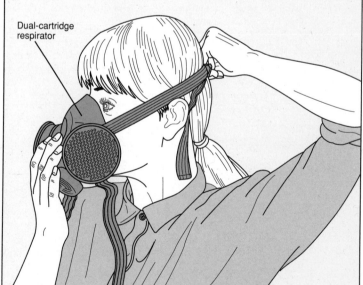

Using respiratory protection. To prevent respiratory problems, wear appropriate respiratory protection to do any dusty work around the house or to use chemicals that emit hazardous vapors. Ensure that any respiratory protection device you use is approved by the National Institute of Occupational Safety and Health (NIOSH). For protection against dust when sanding, drilling or sawing wood, for example, use a dust mask—available at a building supply or home center. For single-use protection, use a disposable dust mask with a sturdy headstrap, a foam seal inside the top and a metal nose clip on the outside *(above, left)*. For repeated-use protection, use a reusable dust mask of rubber with an adjustable headstrap and replaceable cotton or gauze filters. For protection against the hazardous dust of materials such as asbestos, fiberglass or pressure-treated wood, or the hazardous vapors of chemicals marked with POISON vapor and ventilation warnings, use a dual-cartridge respirator *(above, right)*—available at a safety-equipment supply company. Carefully follow the owner's manual instructions for the respirator to install filters or cartridges designed for protection against the particular hazard. Test the respirator before using it; clean and store it properly after using it.

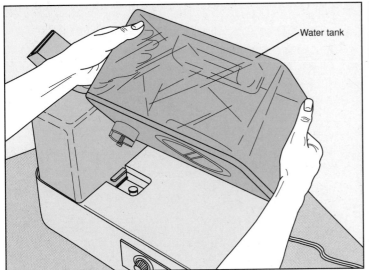

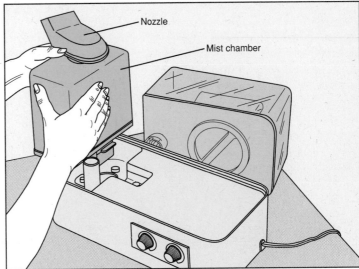

Cleaning a humidifier. Clean a humidifier regularly to prevent the growth and spread of potentially harmful, breathable bacteria. Unplug the humidifier and follow the manufacturer's instructions to disassemble and clean it. For the ultrasonic humidifier shown, remove the water tank *(above, left)*, then the mist chamber and directional nozzle *(above, right)*. Wear rubber gloves to mix a cleaning solution recommended by the humidifier manufacturer. Using a soft, clean cloth dampened with the cleaning solution, gently wash the exterior and interior surfaces of the water tank, the mist chamber, the directional nozzle and any gaskets or covers. Rinse the surfaces thoroughly under running water, then wipe them dry. To clean the reservoir, fill it with your cleaning solution and wait for one hour, then empty it. Use a soft-bristled artist's brush soaked with the cleaning solution to lightly scrub the surfaces of the reservoir, then rinse them thoroughly under running water and wipe them dry. Reassemble the humidifier. Keep any humidifer not in use uncovered.

TREATING AN ALLERGY

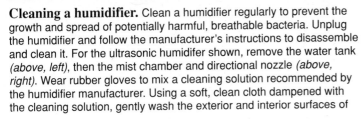

Relieving allergy symptoms. A respiratory allergy is an immune system problem that is characterized by a sudden onset of irritating and sometimes severe respiratory symptoms: sneezing; a runny, stuffy nose; itchy, watering, swollen eyes; an itchy, lumpy skin rash (hives); or, wheezy breathing (asthma).

A person with a respiratory allergy has an immune system that is sensitive to a normally harmless plant or animal substance. When the substance—or allergen—is inhaled through the nose or mouth into the lungs, eaten, or absorbed through the membranes of the eye or a break in the skin, the immune system instantly produces antibodies to attack it. During the process, a chemical called histamine is released into the tissue of the skin, eyes, nose, throat or lungs, producing an allergic reaction within minutes of exposure to the allergen.

Hay fever, or seasonal allergic rhinitis, is the most common respiratory allergy in North America; the allergens that trigger it are the pollens of trees, grasses and weeds, and the spores of molds. Perennial allergic rhinitis occurs on a year-round basis and is triggered by allergens such as dusts, fumes and animal dander.

While there is no "cure" for an allergy, the frequency and severity of an attack can be minimized. To help you manage an allergy, refer to the guidelines below:

• For any severe allergic attack, seek medical help immediately.

• Identify the allergen responsible for any allergic attack. Jot down the time and suspected cause of an attack as well as the nature and severity of the symptoms. Discuss the attack with a physician, asking him about having an allergy test to help pinpoint a difficult-to-identify allergen.

• Reduce exposure to any known allergen. Avoid using fans that can spread allergens around the house. Clean regularly, especially in the bedroom, to minimize dust. Consider using an air-filtration unit or system that is allergy-approved by the Food and Drug Administration (FDA). For hay fever, stay indoors in the morning and on dry, windy days during an allergy season, keeping windows and doors closed; in hot weather, use air conditioning and close any air conditioner vents.

• Avoid using nonprescription allergy-relief medication unless a physician advises it. For a severe allergy symptom, ask a physician to prescribe a medication with few side effects: an oral tablet; drops for the eyes or nose; a nose spray; or a spray inhalant.

• Follow the physician's directions on the prescription label of any medication; use only the amount specified at exactly the prescribed times. Some medications are to be taken only when a symptom develops, while others are to be taken regularly to prevent a symptom from developing.

• Carefully monitor the effects of any prescription medication. Note any side effects or any change in how quickly or well the medication relieves a symptom and report the information to the physician—a different form, dosage or type of medication may be necessary to treat the allergy.

DIGESTIVE SYSTEM

Your digestive system consists of the body organs that break down food so that its nutrients and water can be absorbed into the blood and used by the rest of the body; waste that cannot be absorbed into the blood is expelled by the bowel system. Your urinary system works to expel waste from the blood that cannot be used by the body. The diagram on page 73 illustrates the major organs involved in the body's digestion process.

In the digestive system, food chewed by the teeth passes through the esophagus into the stomach, where stomach acids continue the food breakdown. As the mixture passes through the small intestine, secretions from the pancreas, liver and gallbladder break it down still further so that the nutrients in it can be absorbed through the intestinal wall into the blood for use by the body. Then, as the mixture passes through the colon, the water in it is absorbed into the blood; the dehydrated waste then passes through the rectum and anus to be expelled by a bowel movement. In the urinary system, blood is filtered continuously as it passes through the kidneys; the filtered waste passes in solution through the ureters into the bladder, then through the urethra to be expelled as urine.

Because a myriad of foods and liquids pass through the digestive system every day, minor digestive upsets due to overeating, stress or troublesome bacteria are common. Continual use of the teeth for chewing makes an occasional tooth problem all but inevitable. Similarly, minor urinary tract infections are common, especially in women. The Troubleshooting Guide on pages 74 and 75 puts procedures for common digestive, bowel and urinary ailments at your fingertips, referring you to pages 78 to 83 for more detailed information. Familiarize yourself with the basic techniques for handling an episode of vomiting or diarrhea *(page 78)*, abdominal pain *(page 80)* and indigestion *(page 81)*. An adult with a family history of bowel disease should monitor bowel habits for early warning signs of a potential disorder *(page 81)*. For techniques on handling a life-threatening situation such as poisoning, choking or a diabetic emergency, consult the Emergency Guide *(page 8)*. For basic techniques on caring for a family member who is ill or recuperating from an illness, consult Equipment & Techniques *(page 110)*.

The list of health tips at right covers basic guidelines to help prevent digestive, bowel and urinary ailments—many of which can be avoided with proper tooth care, diet and eating habits, and personal hygiene. As well, annual medical and dental examinations are excellent preventive measures. If you must cope with a digestive, bowel or urinary ailment at home, do not hesitate to call for help; medical professionals can answer questions about symptoms and treatments. Post the telephone numbers for your physician, dentist, local hospital emergency room, poison control center, ambulance and pharmacy near the telephone; in most regions, dial 911 in the event of a life-threatening emergency.

HEALTH TIPS

1. To help prevent the development of a major digestive system disorder, have a thorough medical examination at least once each year; an adult 40 years old or older should request a rectal examination and a stool test to check for occult, or hidden, blood.

2. Prevent minor digestive upsets and long-term digestive disorders by eating a well-balanced diet rich in fiber *(page 76)*. Minimize intake of artificial sweeteners, some of which can cause diarrhea. Minimize intake of sugar which can cause weight problems and tooth decay, and is associated with some types of inflammatory bowel disease.

3. Drink lots of water—8 to 10 glasses per day—and fewer beverages containing sugar or caffeine. Increased water intake reduces the chance of developing urinary tract infections and helps maintain bowel regularity.

4. To aid digestion, get plenty of exercise and fresh air every day—without overdoing it. Walk rather than drive, for example; or, take up a pastime such as swimming, cycling or gardening, choosing an activity to suit your personal tastes and physical strength.

5. Prevent tooth problems that can lead to digestive problems. Care for the teeth properly *(page 76)* and have a dental check-up at least once each year—and the moment you suspect a problem.

6. Prevent minor digestive upsets by making meal times calm and peaceful; chew food slowly and thoroughly. Do not eat while working or driving.

7. Avoid overeating or eating a few large meals each day if you are prone to indigestion; instead, eat more small meals.

8. Unless recommended by your physician, avoid using any nonprescription antacid; some types have high concentrations of salts and other minerals that may have adverse effects. Instead of taking an antacid to help relieve heartburn, drink cold water.

9. Avoid using a nonprescription laxative unless recommended by your physician; some preparations may have adverse effects on the bowels. A physician may recommend a bulk-forming agent such as psyllium seed as a laxative.

10. Follow the physician's directions to use any prescription medication for a digestive or urinary problem; use the amount specified at the prescribed times and report any side effect to the physician.

11. Consult a physician immediately about any potentially-serious symptom of a digestive problem such as vomiting or diarrhea that is prolonged, painful or passes blood—especially in an infant or elderly person.

12. Be aware of any family history of a digestive problem such as a bowel disorder which can be hereditary; an adult at risk for developing a disorder should monitor bowel habits carefully *(page 81)* for early warning signs of a problem.

DIGESTIVE SYSTEM

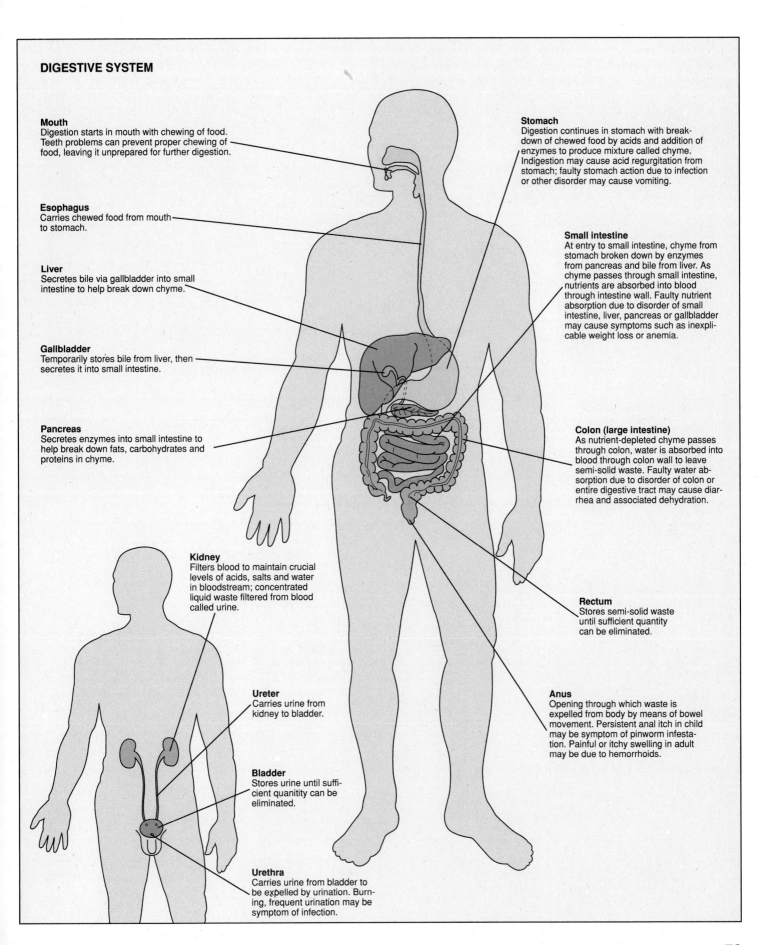

Mouth
Digestion starts in mouth with chewing of food. Teeth problems can prevent proper chewing of food, leaving it unprepared for further digestion.

Esophagus
Carries chewed food from mouth to stomach.

Liver
Secretes bile via gallbladder into small intestine to help break down chyme.

Gallbladder
Temporarily stores bile from liver, then secretes it into small intestine.

Pancreas
Secretes enzymes into small intestine to help break down fats, carbohydrates and proteins in chyme.

Kidney
Filters blood to maintain crucial levels of acids, salts and water in bloodstream; concentrated liquid waste filtered from blood called urine.

Ureter
Carries urine from kidney to bladder.

Bladder
Stores urine until sufficient quanitity can be eliminated.

Urethra
Carries urine from bladder to be expelled by urination. Burning, frequent urination may be symptom of infection.

Stomach
Digestion continues in stomach with break-down of chewed food by acids and addition of enzymes to produce mixture called chyme. Indigestion may cause acid regurgitation from stomach; faulty stomach action due to infection or other disorder may cause vomiting.

Small intestine
At entry to small intestine, chyme from stomach broken down by enzymes from pancreas and bile from liver. As chyme passes through small intestine, nutrients are absorbed into blood through intestine wall. Faulty nutrient absorption due to disorder of small intestine, liver, pancreas or gallbladder may cause symptoms such as inexplicable weight loss or anemia.

Colon (large intestine)
As nutrient-depleted chyme passes through colon, water is absorbed into blood through colon wall to leave semi-solid waste. Faulty water absorption due to disorder of colon or entire digestive tract may cause diarrhea and associated dehydration.

Rectum
Stores semi-solid waste until sufficient quantity can be eliminated.

Anus
Opening through which waste is expelled from body by means of bowel movement. Persistent anal itch in child may be symptom of pinworm infestation. Painful or itchy swelling in adult may be due to hemorrhoids.

TROUBLESHOOTING GUIDE

PROBLEM	PROCEDURE
Toothache	If pain severe, use a nonprescription pain-reliever *(p. 121)*
	Consult a dentist to treat tooth
	Care for teeth *(p. 76)*
Tooth broken	Treat broken tooth *(p. 82)*
	Consult a dentist immediately to treat tooth
Teeth yellow, stained	Consult a dentist to clean teeth
	Care for teeth *(p. 76)*
Gum red, swollen or tender; bleeds easily	Consult a dentist to treat gums
	Care for teeth *(p. 76)*
Mouth or lip sore	Treat mouth or lip sore *(p. 82)*
	Care for teeth *(p. 76)*
	Consult a physician if sore does not heal in 5 days
Appetite loss or refusal to eat (infant or child)	Provide rest; fluids
	Watch for and treat any secondary problem
	Consult a physician if appetite loss or refusal to eat lasts more than 1 day
Appetite loss (adolescent or adult)	Rest; minimize stress; drink fluids
	Watch for and treat any secondary problem
	Consult a physician if appetite loss lasts more than 1 week
Weight loss unexplained (infant or child)	Consult a physician
Weight loss unexplained (adolescent)	Watch for and treat any emotional disorder *(p. 48)*
	Watch for and treat any secondary problem
	Consult a physician if weight loss lasts more than 1 month
Weight loss unexplained (adult)	Monitor bowel habits *(p. 81)*
	Watch for and treat any secondary problem
	Consult a physician if weight loss lasts more than 1 month
Weight gain unexplained	Monitor bowel habits *(p. 81)*
	Watch for and treat any secondary problem
	Consult a physician if weight gain lasts more than 3 months
Constipation: difficult, infrequent bowel movements	Use a non-prescription laxative only if recommended by physician
	Maintain balanced diet *(p. 76)*; drink plenty of fluids, exercise and minimize stress
	Monitor bowel habits *(p. 81)*
	Watch for and treat any secondary problem
	Consult a physician if there is no bowel movement for more than 3 days, constipation lasts more than 2 weeks or mild episodes of constipation become chronic
Diarrhea: loose, frequent bowel movements	Seek emergency help ✚ if diarrhea severe or accompanied by bleeding, severe abdominal pain or severe vomiting
	Consult a physician if diarrhea follows trip to foreign country or affects infant or elderly person
	Use a nonprescription diarrhea remedy only if recommended by physician
	Treat diarrhea *(p. 78)*
	Watch for and treat any secondary problem
	Consult a physician if diarrhea lasts more than 2 days (more than 12 hours in an infant) or mild episodes of diarrhea become chronic
Stools discolored: red or black and tarry	Consult a physician
Family history of bowel disease	Monitor bowel habits *(p. 81)*

✚ Medical emergency

TROUBLESHOOTING GUIDE

PROBLEM	PROCEDURE
Hemorrhoids suspected: itchy or painful anal swelling	Wash anal area thoroughly after bowel movements
	Sit in warm bath for 10 to 20 minutes as often as possible
	Maintain balanced diet *(p. 76)*; drink plenty of fluids, exercise and minimize stress
	Consult a physician if anal discomfort persistent, bowel movements painful or blood passed with stools
Pinworms suspected: child suffers persistent anal itch	Treat pinworms *(p. 79)*
Vomiting	Seek emergency help ✚ if vomiting severe or accompanied by bleeding (vomit has appearance of coffee grounds), severe abdominal pain or severe diarrhea
	Treat vomiting *(p. 78)*
	Watch for and treat any secondary problem
	Consult a physician if vomiting lasts more than 4 hours or mild episodes of vomiting become chronic
Abdominal pain	Seek emergency help ✚ if abdominal pain severe, accompanied by severe vomiting or severe diarrhea, or occurs during pregnancy
	Treat abdominal pain *(p. 80)*
	Watch for and treat any secondary problem
	Consult a physician if abdominal pain worsens or persists without change for more than 3 hours or mild episodes of abdominal pain become chronic
Indigestion suspected: burping, gas, hiccups, acid regurgitation or heartburn after eating	Seek emergency help ✚ if burning chest pain radiates to jaw, neck or arm and accompanied by sweating, nausea, dizziness or shortness of breath
	Use a nonprescription antacid only if recommended by physician
	Treat indigestion *(p. 81)*
	Consult a physician if indigestion severe or if episodes of indigestion become chronic
Heartburn suspected: burning sensation in upper abdomen after eating	Seek emergency help ✚ if burning chest pain radiates to jaw, neck or arm and accompanied by sweating, nausea, dizziness or shortness of breath
	Use a nonprescription antacid only if recommended by physician
	Treat indigestion *(p. 81)*
	Consult a physician if heartburn severe or if episodes of heartburn become chronic
Urination frequent	Reduce consumption of liquids—especially beverages of alcohol and caffeine
	Watch for and treat any secondary problem
	Consult a physician if frequent urination interrupts daily routines or sleeping habits
Urination painful, burning	Consult a physician
	If necessary, treat urinary tract infection *(p. 83)*
Urinary control loss	Consult a physician
Urination inability	Consult a physician if inability to urinate lasts more than 24 hours
Urine discolored: red or dark	Consult a physician

✚ Medical emergency

MAINTAINING A BALANCED DIET

Following a fiber-rich diet. If you have a disorder of the digestive tract, discuss any change in your intake of dietary fiber with your doctor. Most medical experts agree that the average individual in the U.S. eats too little fiber. Susceptibility to constipation, hemorrhoids and other digestive problems may be reduced with an adequate intake of fiber; meanwhile, new studies suggest that a fiber-rich diet may benefit overall health much more than previously thought. Also, the intake of more fiber and less fat is advised to help prevent cancer of the colon. Although opinions can differ on the amount of fiber that should be included in the diet of an individual, an adult is usually advised to consume about 35 grams of fiber daily.

To calculate your daily intake of fiber, consult the chart at right. If your daily intake of fiber is less than 35 grams, you can increase it to this level by 5 to 10 grams per day over one week—also adding to your intake of water. A rapid increase in the intake of fiber can cause bloating and cramps. Gradually add fiber to your diet by eating whole grain breads instead of refined white breads, for example. Include one or two tablespoons of bran with refined commercial cereals to boost their fiber content. Replace calorie-laden desserts with fruit, adding other important nutrients along with fiber to your diet. Cut down on your intake of meat, substituting it with dried beans or lentils—both rich in fiber and protein. Eat a variety of fiber-rich foods; do not rely on a single food to provide the requisite daily amount of fiber.

FOOD	AMOUNT	FIBER
Kidney, navy or pinto beans; cooked and dried	1 cup	12 grams
100% bran flakes	3/4 cup	12 grams
Peas or soybeans; cooked and dried	1 cup	8 grams
Parsnips; cooked and dried	3/4 cup	6 grams
Grapefruit	1 medium	5 grams
Broccoli, carrots or zucchini; cooked and dried	1 cup	4 grams
Corn kernels; cooked and dried	2/3 cup	4 grams
40% bran flakes with raisins	3/4 cup	4 grams
Apple or pear; with skin	1 medium	3 grams
Wheat germ	1/2 cup	2 to 3 grams
Strawberries	1/2 cup	2 to 3 grams
Potato; with skin	1 medium	2 grams
Dates	4 medium	2 grams
Buckwheat	2 tablespoons	2 grams
Cabbage; cooked and dried	3/4 cup	2 grams
Beets; cooked and dried	2/3 cup	2 grams
Celery; raw	2 medium stalks	2 grams
Spinach; raw	2 large leaves	2 grams
Bread; 100% whole wheat, rye or pumpernickel	1 slice	1 to 2 grams
Brown rice; cooked	1 cup	1 gram

CARING FOR THE TEETH: ADULTS

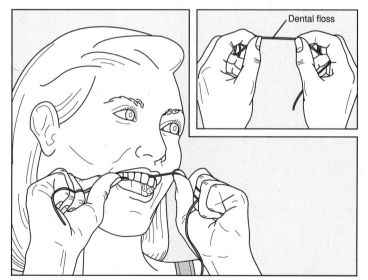

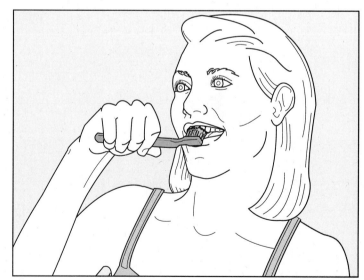

1 **Flossing the teeth.** Floss your teeth at least once each day, preferably just before you brush them. Break off about 18 inches of dental floss and wind one end of it loosely around the middle finger of one hand, leaving about 12 inches of it free to hold with your other hand *(inset)*. Guiding the floss carefully between two adjacent teeth, use a gentle back-and-forth sawing motion to scrape the surface of each adjacent tooth, removing food particles and plaque; continue until just below the gum line *(above)*. Floss between each pair of adjacent teeth the same way, unwinding or breaking off more floss to use a clean length of it. If desired, a small device for holding the floss can be purchased at a pharmacy.

2 **Brushing the teeth.** Brush your teeth at least twice each day using a fluoride toothpaste. Unless your dentist recommends a specific toothbrush for your teeth, choose a soft-bristled type that is small enough for you to reach the entire surface of each tooth. Holding the toothbrush at about a 45-degree angle to the teeth, brush thoroughly to remove plaque using the technique recommended by your dentist or dental hygienist; be sure to brush both the outer *(above)* and inner surfaces of each tooth. To further reduce bacterial build-up in the mouth, use your toothbrush to gently brush the top surface of your tongue. Rinse your mouth well with water.

CARING FOR THE TEETH: INFANTS AND CHILDREN

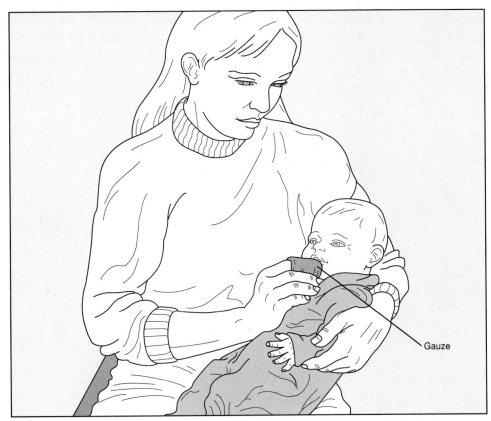

Gauze

Taking care of an infant's gums and teeth. When an infant begins to eat solid food, you should clean his gums and any teeth at least once each day. Wash your hands thoroughly with soap and water, then wipe them dry using a clean towel. Seat the infant on your lap, cradling him in your arms with his head supported securely against your chest. Dampen a small piece of sterile gauze with water and hold it over your index finger. Carefully work your index finger into the infant's mouth, gently rubbing the dampened gauze over his gums *(left)* and any teeth. Consult your dentist about the age that the infant should reach before you apply the same technique with toothpaste. You may be advised against using a fluoride toothpaste with an infant if the water supply in your area is fluoridated, or you administer fluoridated vitamins or other fluoride preparations.

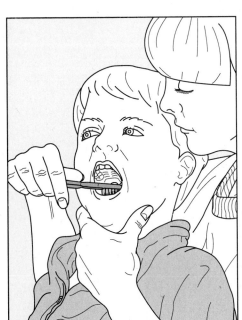

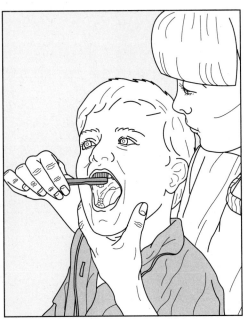

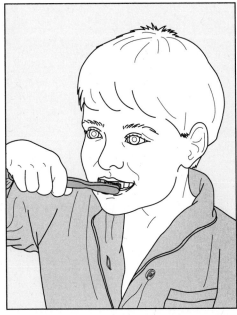

Taking care of a child's teeth. Once a child has all his teeth, brush them at least twice each day using a fluoride toothpaste. Unless your dentist recommends a specific toothbrush, choose a soft-bristled type that is small enough to reach the entire surface of each of the child's teeth. Seat or stand the child at a sink. Resting the child's head comfortably against your shoulder with one hand supporting his chin, have the child open his mouth wide. Holding the toothbrush at 45-degree angle to the child's teeth, brush thoroughly to remove plaque using the technique recommended by your dentist or dental hygienist. Be sure to brush both the outer and inner surfaces of the lower teeth *(above, left)* and the upper teeth *(above, center)*. Have the child rinse his mouth with water. Once the child can handle a toothbrush, carefully supervise him as he brushes his teeth himself *(above, right)*. Check the thoroughness of the child's brushing using disclosing tablets, available at a pharmacy. Follow the manufacturer's instructions to administer a tablet to the child, then inspect his teeth for traces of dye that mark remaining plaque; have the child brush again to remove any dye. Consult your dentist about the age that the child should reach before he flosses and brushes his teeth as an adult *(page 76)*.

TREATING VOMITING AND DIARRHEA

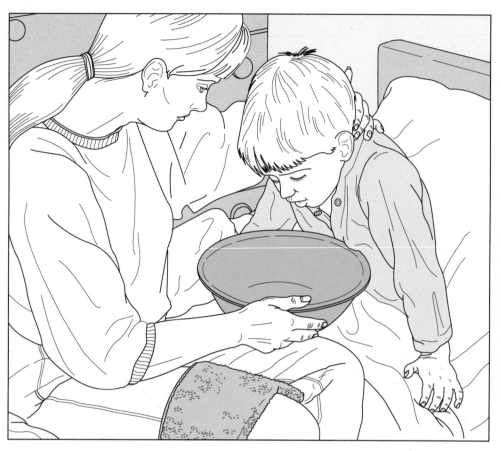

1 Caring for a sick person. Vomiting and diarrhea are common digestive upsets caused by infection, food poisoning, a food allergy, stress or overeating. For diarrhea in an infant or elderly person, or following a trip abroad, consult a physician. Otherwise, treat any episode of vomiting or diarrhea the same way. Stop all eating and drink only water: occasional sips for vomiting; as much as can be tolerated for diarrhea. Have a sick person rest in bed or sitting down. To care for a child who may be frightened by an episode of vomiting or diarrhea, stay nearby and hold him securely to provide reassurance *(left)*; then, gently wipe his face with a warm cloth. After vomiting, have the child rinse his mouth with water; after an episode of diarrhea, clean him thoroughly, if necessary. Consult a physician if: an episode is severe; there is severe abdominal pain; water intake cannot be tolerated; vomit or diarrhea contains blood; vomiting continues for more than 4 hours; or diarrhea persists for more than 2 days—12 hours with an infant. Also consult a physician if a child stops urinating for more than 8 hours; with an adult, for more than 12 hours. When the vomiting or diarrhea has passed, replace lost fluids and introduce food gradually *(step 2)*.

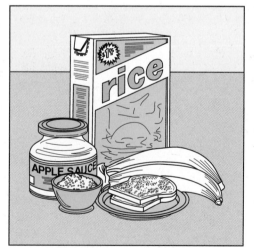

2 Replacing lost fluids. Once the vomiting or diarrhea has passed, replace lost fluids for about 6 hours before reintroducing solid food. Avoid giving a sick person a milk product, which can be difficult to digest, or a drink with a high sugar content, which can act as a laxative. Have the person drink water, taking small sips at frequent intervals. Or, prepare and administer an easy-to-digest electrolyte solution that approximates the mineral balance of the body's own fluids. Buy a commercially-formulated electrolyte solution at a pharmacy and follow the manufacturer's instructions on the label to administer it. Alternatively, prepare your own electrolyte solution by mixing 1 teaspoon of salt, 1 teaspoon of baking soda (sodium bicarbonate) and 4 teaspoons of sugar per quart of water; if desired, add 2 to 4 tablespoons of apple juice for flavor. Then, have the person drink the solution, taking small sips at frequent intervals. Once the person has replaced lost fluids, begin a gradual reintroduction of solid food. Start with small amounts of easy-to-digest foods such as banana, rice, applesauce and dry toast *(right)*. Then, once the person feels well enough, reintroduce other foods in larger quantities; avoid any intake of fatty or sugary foods until the person is fully recuperated.

Preventing diarrhea. To prevent the spread of an infection that causes diarrhea, practice good hygiene; always wash the hands thoroughly after using the toilet. To prevent food contamination that can cause diarrhea, always use proper food-handling techniques *(page 79)*. If a family member has had diarrhea, take extra precautions to prevent the spread of it within the household. Wash the hands thoroughly after handling or changing an infant or child affected by diarrhea; wash the clothing and bedding of a person affected by diarrhea separately from other laundry.

Take special precautions to prevent diarrhea when traveling abroad, especially to an area that may have a contaminated water supply. Before leaving the country, ask your physician for a prescription for a diarrhea medication; as an added protection, also take along a supply of a commercially-formulated electrolyte solution to help replace lost fluids in the event of an episode of diarrhea *(step 2, above)*. While abroad, avoid eating raw foods, unpasteurized dairy products or unpeeled fruit, and avoid drinking tap water or using ice made from tap water.

TREATING PINWORMS

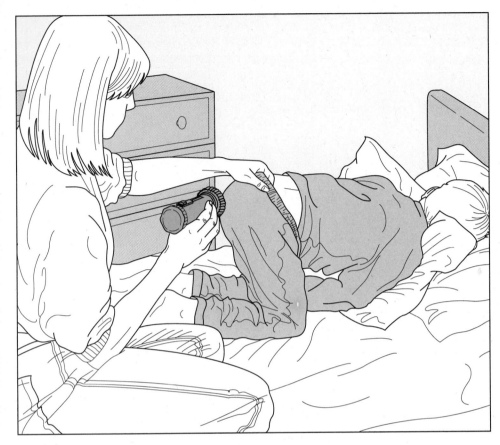

Caring for the child. A child who has a persistently-itchy anus may have pinworms. To inspect a child for pinworms, work at night in a dark room. Have the child position himself comfortably, then use a flashlight *(left)* to examine his anus; any tiny lint-like organisms that move in the light are pinworms. To treat pinworms, consult your physician for an appropriate medication. Use the medication for the length of time specified by the physician, following the directions on the label to use the amount specified at the prescribed times. To prevent a pinworm reinfestation, wash all clothing, bedding and linen used by the child with laundry bleach and boiling water. Vacuum and clean the child's mattress and box spring, wash all his toys, and discard any modeling clay. Have the child practice proper hygiene; keep his fingernails short and clean, and ensure that he washes his hands after using the toilet and before eating. Have any family pet examined by a veterinarian to determine if pinworms are being carried by it. Prevent any food contamination that can cause pinworms by handling food properly *(step below)*.

PREVENTING FOOD CONTAMINATION

Handling food properly. Always store, prepare and cook food properly to help prevent contamination by bacteria that can cause the vomiting and diarrhea associated with food poisoning, or by parasites such as pinworms. The bacteria that can cause food poisoning are present in the air, water and soil, as well as on the skin and in the intestinal tracts of household pets and the animals we eat as meat. Consuming small amounts of these bacteria usually poses little danger, but if food is carelessly stored and prepared or improperly cooked, these bacteria may become active and multiply in large quantities. Refer to the guidelines below for suggestions about handling food properly and preventing contamination that can cause digestive system disorders:

• Refrigerate food that must be kept cold as quickly as possible after buying it; never refrigerate partially-cooked meat.

• Set a refrigerator thermostat no higher than 40° Fahrenheit.

• Discard any food if it smells or looks odd, or if its container bulges or leaks or is moldy on the inside.

• Thaw food in the refrigerator or in a plastic bag in cold water. Cook food thawed in a microwave oven immediately.

• Wash your hands before and after handling raw meat, poultry, seafood or eggs.

• Wash any utensil or kitchen surface that has been in contact with raw meat, poultry or seafood using hot, soapy water.

• Always use clean towels to dry your hands and cooking utensils.

• Regularly clean a cutting board using a solution of 1 part laundry bleach to 16 parts water, rinsing it thoroughly.

• Keep the kitchen free of flying and crawling insects.

• Wash fruits and vegetables to remove any soil and pesticide.

• Stuff poultry only immediately before cooking it; remove stuffing from poultry before refrigerating it.

• Use a meat thermometer to ensure that a meat is cooked to the correct internal temperature: 160° Fahrenheit for pork; 170° Fahrenheit for poultry; and 165° Fahrenheit for any stuffing.

• Heat leftovers to an internal temperature of 165° Fahrenheit.

• Never let any food that has been cooked or that must be refrigerated stand at room temperature more than 4 hours.

TREATING ABDOMINAL PAIN

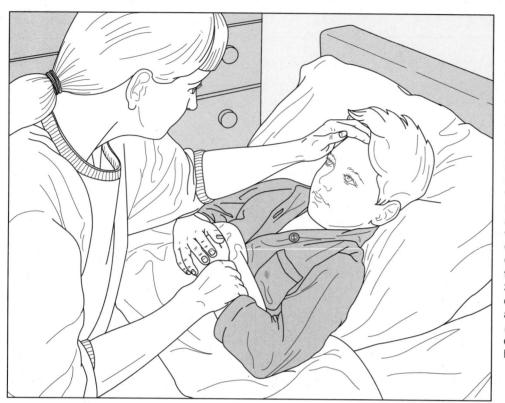

Relieving abdominal pain in a child or adult. Abdominal pain, especially in a child, is a common digestive upset that may be caused by an infection, food poisoning, stress or overeating. Consult a physician if abdominal pain is severe, especially if a child is wakened or cannot sleep with it. Otherwise, stop all eating, drink only water and rest in bed; to treat a child, stay nearby to provide reassurance *(left)*. Avoid using any treatment for the pain that might mask the symptoms of a serious problem—appendicitis in a child, for example. Do not: apply an ice pack or a hot-water bottle on the abdomen; use a pain-reliever; or, use a laxative, a suppository or an enema. If necessary, treat any episode of vomiting or diarrhea *(page 78)* that occurs. Otherwise, continue to monitor the situation. Consult a physician as soon as possible if: the pain worsens or persists for longer than 3 hours; the pain is aggravated by movement or pressure on the abdomen; the abdomen appears distended; or, there is a high fever *(page 114)*. Do not hesitate to consult a physician if you are worried, especially if a child has had previous episodes of abdominal pain.

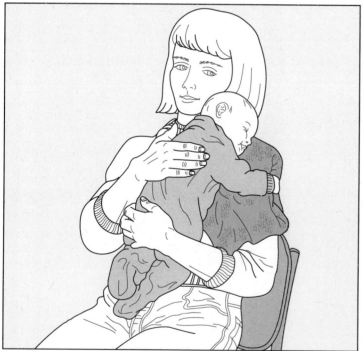

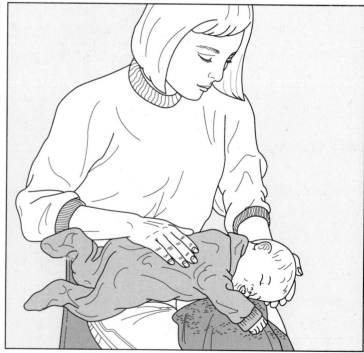

Relieving abdominal pain in an infant. An infant that cries and draws up its legs has abdominal pain; an episode during or soon after feeding is normal and is usually a sign of gas—a result of the infant swallowing air while feeding. Whenever you suspect that an infant has gas, relieve the discomfort; prevent abdominal pain by relieving gas at least once during each feeding and once after it. Pick up the infant and hold him upright against your shoulder *(above, left)*; or, lay the infant on his stomach on your lap and firmly support this head *(above, right)*. Then, gently pat and rub the infant's back until any gas is passed. Consult a physician about any abdominal pain in an infant that seems severe, frequent or long-lasting, or that is characterized by extreme and unconsolable crying.

TREATING INDIGESTION

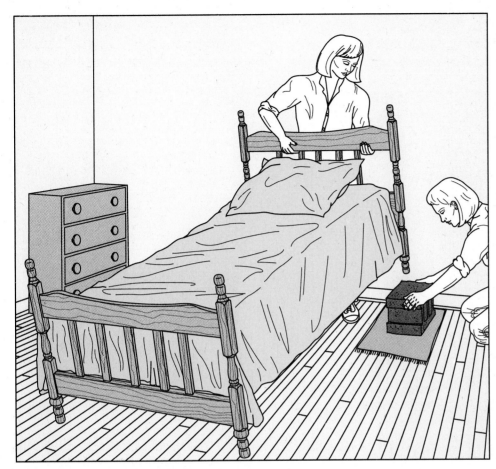

Relieving indigestion. Digestive discomfort following eating is common in many adults, especially pregnant women. The typical symptoms of indigestion include a bloated-feeling stomach, burping, gas, hiccups, stomach acid regurgitation and a burning sensation in the upper abdomen (heartburn). **Caution:** Burning chest pain radiating to the jaw, neck or arm that is accompanied by sweating, nausea, dizziness or shortness of breath may be signs of a heart problem requiring emergency help *(page 8)*. To treat indigestion, avoid using a nonprescription antacid unless your physician recommends it; instead, modify your eating habits and lifestyle. Regulate your food intake by eating frequent, small meals; if you are overweight, consult your physician about losing weight. Avoid foods and substances that aggravate indigestion: coffee, chocolate, fried or fatty foods, alcohol, aspirin, and tobacco smoke, for example. Avoid strenuous exercise or bending immediately after eating. During bowel movements, avoid straining. To minimize discomfort from indigestion during sleep, raise the head of the bed 4 to 6 inches by propping up the legs *(left)*. For severe or frequent indigestion that does not respond to self-help, consult your physician.

MONITORING BOWEL HABITS

Detecting early warning signs of cancer. Research done by the American Cancer Society indicates that colorectal (colon and rectum) cancer is the second leading cause of cancer-related deaths in the United States. Persons most at risk for the development of colorectal cancer typically have a family history of colorectal cancer, polyps or an inflammatory bowel disease such as ulcerative colitis. If you are 35 years old or older, you should take steps to prevent the development of colorectal cancer—especially if you are at high risk. Monitor your habits carefully to help you detect any early warning signs of colorectal cancer or other major disease:

• **Maintaining a balanced diet.** Although no precise relationship has been established between diet and colorectal cancer, some studies indicate that a diet too high in fat and too low in fiber may contribute to its development—particularly among those with a family history of bowel disease. In general, maintain a balanced diet that is low in fat and high in fiber *(page 76)*.

• **Monitoring bowel habits.** Be alert to the early warning signs of a possible bowel disease. Watch closely for any unusual and persistent changes in your bowel habits. Consult a physician if: occasional episodes of diarrhea or constipation become chronic or you have alternating episodes of diarrhea and constipation; your stools contain blood or mucus or become pencil-thin or flat and ribbon-like; you experience any rectal bleeding; you have non-specific abdominal pains and cramps that become chronic; you experience any unexplained weight loss, anemia or on-going, general malaise.

• **Having a rectal examination.** A person 40 years old or older should have an annual rectal examination; consult a physician to arrange it. For a digital examination, the physician inserts a finger through the anus into the rectum to feel for any abnormality. If you are 50 years old or older, the physician may recommend a proctosigmoidoscopy; for this examination, the physician inserts a hollow, lighted tube through the anus and rectum into the colon to look for any abnormality.

• **Having a stool test.** A person 40 years old or older should have an annual stool test to check for hidden blood that may indicate a colon problem. Although home-testing kits are available, it is best to consult a physician for a stool test to ensure that proper procedures are followed—especially if you have hemorrhoids or are menstruating. Be sure that you maintain the dietary restrictions required for the 2 to 3 days of the test period; also maintain any other restrictions required scrupulously.

TREATING A BROKEN TOOTH

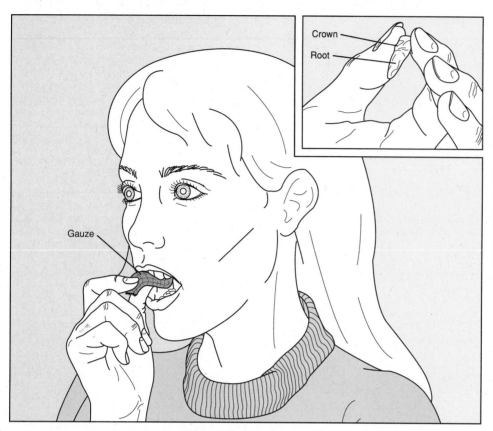

Preserving a tooth. If a severe impact loosens, breaks or knocks out a tooth, take quick steps to stop any bleeding and preserve the tooth, if possible; then, consult a dentist immediately. To stop any bleeding, position a pad of sterile gauze over the loose or broken tooth or the socket in the gum and bite down on it to hold it in place *(left)*. If a knocked-out tooth remains intact, preserve it. Carefully pick up the tooth by its crown—never its root *(inset)*. If the tooth is clean and the gum is not bleeding severely, carefully reinsert the root of the tooth into the socket of the gum and hold it in place using a pad of sterile gauze. Otherwise, preserve the tooth for up to 12 hours by placing it in an emergency tooth-preserving system *(page 110)* or a tightly-sealed jar of cold milk. Do not place the tooth in water or clean it with a disinfectant; any live cells can be killed.

TREATING A MOUTH OR LIP SORE

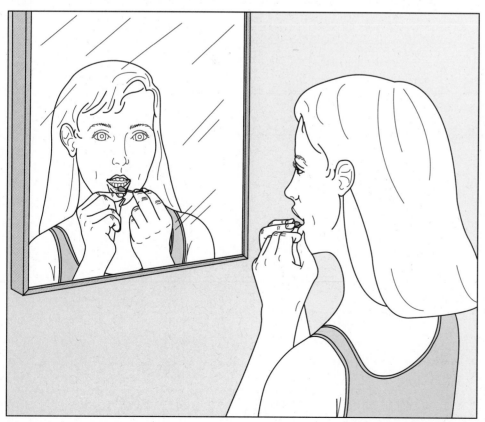

Treating a sore. A mouth or lip sore is a common problem, especially among children, and is usually due to a minor infection that clears up within a few days. To minimize discomfort from a mouth or lip sore, avoid eating or drinking salty or acidic substances that can irritate the sore. Periodically rinse the mouth with warm water to wash the sore; for minor pain, use a nonprescription pain-reliever *(page 121)*. To speed the healing of a sore, buy an antiseptic nonprescription ointment for it at a pharmacy. Follow the manufacturer's instructions to apply the ointment, using a clean cotton swab to gently dab it onto the sore *(left)*. To prevent the sore from becoming infected, avoid touching it with your hands. To keep a contagious sore from spreading, wash your hands thoroughly after applying any ointment; do not share eating utensils, drinking glasses, towels or facecloths. Consult a physician for a mouth or lip sore that does not heal within 5 days or if mouth and lip sores are recurrent.

TREATING A URINARY TRACT INFECTION

Relieving and preventing minor infections. Minor urinary tract infections are common among adults, especially women, and are usually not cause for serious concern. The typical symptoms of a minor infection include a burning or painful sensation during urination and frequent urination. Other accompanying symptoms, however, may indicate a more serious problem. Consult a physician if: pain is severe; there is any discharge from the urinary tract; urine is dark and discolored; there is an inability to hold urine; or, there is an inability to urinate for longer than 1 day. Otherwise, if you are in good health, treat a minor urinary tract infection yourself for 48 hours to try and clear it up; eliminate coffee and alcohol, and drink enough water to urinate fully once each hour. If the infection persists, consult a physician; if requested, collect a urine sample *(step below)* to bring to the consultation. Refer to the guidelines below to treat a diagnosed, minor urinary tract infection and help prevent an annoying recurrence:

• Follow the physician's directions to use any prescription medication for the infection; take the amount specified at the prescribed times and report any side effect to the physician.

• Relieve the soreness and discomfort of an infection by using a nonprescription pain-reliever *(page 121)*.

• To avoid aggravating an infection, eliminate coffee, alcohol or other drinks and any food that adds to your discomfort.

• To keep from aggravating an infection, avoid using scented soaps, deodorant sprays and colored toilet paper.

• Minimize the duration of an infection by drinking enough water to urinate fully every hour. Avoid holding urine; urinate as soon as you feel the need, emptying the bladder completely.

• To help prevent an infection, wear cotton undergarments and change to fresh undergarments daily.

• To help prevent an infection, thoroughly clean the genital area after urination and the rectal area after a bowel movement; a female should always clean from front to back.

• Help prevent an infection by thoroughly washing the genital area daily; a female should wash from front to back and an uncircumcised male should clean beneath the foreskin.

• To help avoid an infection, a female should change hygienic pads frequently and thoroughly wash the genital area twice daily during menstruation.

• Help prevent an infection, by thoroughly washing the genital area before sexual intercourse. Urinate and thoroughly wash the genital area again after sexual intercourse.

• Make the necessary effort to help maintain the body's resistance to an infection by eating and sleeping properly, and avoiding stress as much as possible.

COLLECTING A URINE SAMPLE

Collecting a urine sample. To assist in the diagnosis of a urinary tract infection or other condition, a physician may request that a urine sample be collected at home and brought to a consultation. Have the physician explain how to collect the sample; it may need to be taken at a specified time of day, or within a specified time before or after eating or drinking, for example. In general, you are likely to be asked for a "clean-catch, mid-stream" urine sample—collected after some urine has passed, that is as free as possible from contaminants. For a female who is menstruating, the physician may recommend inserting a tampon for the collection of a urine sample.

Collect the urine sample no more than 24 hours before you are scheduled to see the physician. Use a small, clean glass jar with a tight-fitting lid and have on hand a supply of clean cotton balls *(right)* or, if recommended by the physician, antiseptic towellettes. Wash your hands, then use a cotton ball soaked in warm water or an antiseptic towellette to clean the urethral opening. For a male, retract any foreskin and wipe one way across the tip of the penis. For a female, clean the edge of the urethral opening by wiping one way from front to back. Begin urinating in the toilet. Without interrupting the flow of urine, position the jar to catch it. Fill the jar partway with urine, then remove it before the flow of urine stops and finish urinating in the toilet. Without touching the rim or the inside of the jar or the inside of the lid, close the jar and wipe the outside of it clean. Label the jar "urine" and place it in a container or plastic bag. Wash your hands thoroughly, then place the container or plastic bag in the refrigerator away from food until you are ready to go to see your physician.

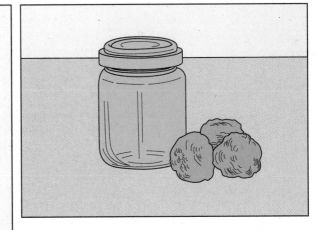

REPRODUCTIVE SYSTEM

Your reproductive system includes the parts of the body involved in reproduction that provide you with your unique anatomical and hormonal characteristics as a female or a male. The diagrams on page 85 illustrate the major organs of the reproductive system of a typical female and a typical male.

In the female, the ovaries produce ova that are released monthly to the fallopian tubes and uterus; the ova are either fertilized by male sperm and implanted in the uterus during pregnancy or expelled with the uterine lining through the vagina during menstruation. As part of the endocrine system, the ovaries produce and secrete the female hormones estrogen and progesterone to stimulate breast and hair development as well as menstruation during adolescence, and to regulate menstruation during adulthood.

In the male, the testicles produce sperm that are stored in the vas deferens and seminal vesicles, then mixed with seminal fluid from the prostate gland and expelled through the urethra from the penis during ejaculation. As part of the endocrine system, the testicles produce and secrete the male hormone testosterone to stimulate hair and genital development as well as voice changes during adolescence, and to maintain these characteristics during adulthood.

Disorders of the reproductive system are not common household medical problems and can usually be avoided with proper preventive care. The health tips at right provide guidelines for helping to maintain a properly-functioning reproductive system. Always use proper genital and sexual hygiene practices *(page 91)* to prevent the development of genital irritations and infections. To help detect the early warning signs of cancer or any other abnormality, an adult female should perform a monthly breast self-examination *(page 88)* and an adult male should perform a monthly testicle self-examination *(page 89)*. Regular medical examinations by a physician are also excellent preventive measures; an adult female should have a periodic breast and cervical examination, and any male over 40 years of age should request an annual prostate gland examination and be alert to the signs of a possible prostate gland disorder *(page 90)*. Family members should also be alert to important changes and possible problems of the reproductive system that occur during pregnancy *(page 87)* and puberty *(page 89)*.

The Troubleshooting Guide *(page 86)* puts procedures for dealing with reproductive system problems at your fingertips. In the event of any life-threatening emergency, use the Emergency Guide *(page 8)*. For techniques on caring for a family member who is ill or recuperating from an illness, consult the Equipment & Techniques chapter *(page 110)*. If you must cope with a reproductive system problem in the home, do not hesitate to call for help; medical professionals can answer questions about symptoms and treatments. Post the telephone numbers for your physician, local hospital emergency room, ambulance and pharmacy near the telephone; in most regions, dial 911 in a life-threatening emergency.

HEALTH TIPS

1. To prevent minor genital irritations and infections, practice proper genital hygiene *(page 91)*. In general, avoid applying a scented soap or any deodorant or perfume to the genital area; many commercial bubble bath products, for example, can cause irritation, especially in a child.

2. To help prevent vaginal infections and odors, change tampons or hygienic napkins frequently during menstruation; avoid leaving a tampon inserted for more than 3 hours.

3. To help prevent vaginal infections, a woman should wipe from front to back after any bowel movement, preventing the entry of infectious bacteria into the vagina.

4. A woman should consult a physician about any unusual change in menstrual patterns such as an unexplained absence of a period, any suddenly or increasingly painful periods, or any suddenly or increasingly heavier periods.

5. Cervical cancer is becoming an increasingly common form of cancer among young women. A woman 20 years of age or older should talk to her physician about undergoing a smear test regularly to help detect the early warning signs of a possible cervical disorder.

6. Breast cancer is a major cause of cancer-related deaths among women 35 years of age and older. To help detect the early warning signs of a breast abnormality, a woman 20 years of age or older should perform a breast self-examination monthly *(page 88)*. A woman 20 to 40 years of age should also have a breast examination by a physician every 3 years; a woman over 40 years of age should have one annually.

7. Be alert to the warning signs of a possible problem during pregnancy *(page 87)*. Consult a physician immediately if there is breathlessness during the first trimester or at rest, nausea or vomiting after the first trimester, vaginal bleeding at any time, a weight gain of more than 4 pounds in one week, or a weight loss of more than 2 pounds in one week.

8. Testicular cancer is the most common cancer among men between 18 and 35 years of age, but can often be cured if it is detected and treated early. To help detect the early warning signs of a testicle abnormality, a man 20 years of age or older should perform a testicle self-examination monthly *(page 89)*.

9. To help detect the early warning signs of a prostate gland disorder, men 40 years of age and older should have a rectal examination as part of an annual medical checkup.

10. Familiarize yourself with the typical patterns of adolescent sexual development during puberty and be prepared to assist an adolescent making the transition to adulthood *(page 90)*. If necessary, consult a physician about any physical or emotional problems during the puberty of an adolescent.

11. Be alert to the symptoms of a sexually-transmitted disease as well as the appropriate strategy for managing and preventing the transmission of sexually-transmitted diseases *(page 91)*; consult a physician about any urethral discharge or any sore, rash, itchiness or pain in the genital area.

FEMALE REPRODUCTIVE SYSTEM

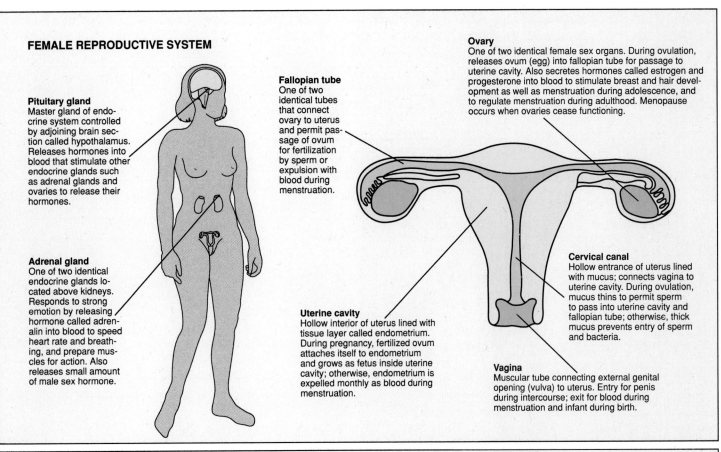

Pituitary gland
Master gland of endocrine system controlled by adjoining brain section called hypothalamus. Releases hormones into blood that stimulate other endocrine glands such as adrenal glands and ovaries to release their hormones.

Adrenal gland
One of two identical endocrine glands located above kidneys. Responds to strong emotion by releasing hormone called adrenalin into blood to speed heart rate and breathing, and prepare muscles for action. Also releases small amount of male sex hormone.

Fallopian tube
One of two identical tubes that connect ovary to uterus and permit passage of ovum for fertilization by sperm or expulsion with blood during menstruation.

Uterine cavity
Hollow interior of uterus lined with tissue layer called endometrium. During pregnancy, fertilized ovum attaches itself to endometrium and grows as fetus inside uterine cavity; otherwise, endometrium is expelled monthly as blood during menstruation.

Ovary
One of two identical female sex organs. During ovulation, releases ovum (egg) into fallopian tube for passage to uterine cavity. Also secretes hormones called estrogen and progesterone into blood to stimulate breast and hair development as well as menstruation during adolescence, and to regulate menstruation during adulthood. Menopause occurs when ovaries cease functioning.

Cervical canal
Hollow entrance of uterus lined with mucus; connects vagina to uterine cavity. During ovulation, mucus thins to permit sperm to pass into uterine cavity and fallopian tube; otherwise, thick mucus prevents entry of sperm and bacteria.

Vagina
Muscular tube connecting external genital opening (vulva) to uterus. Entry for penis during intercourse; exit for blood during menstruation and infant during birth.

MALE REPRODUCTIVE SYSTEM

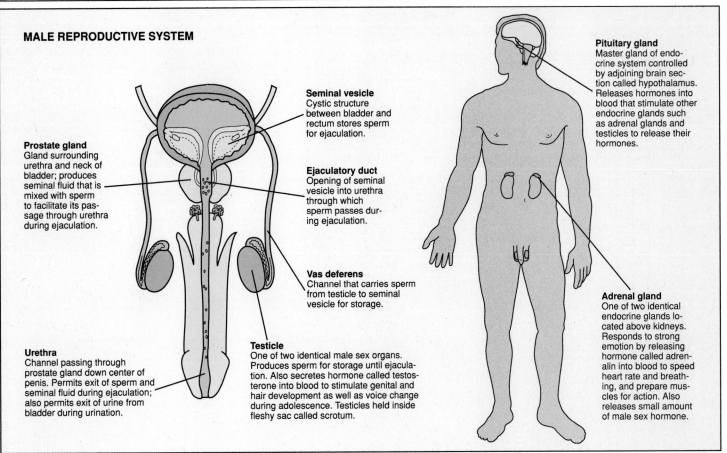

Prostate gland
Gland surrounding urethra and neck of bladder; produces seminal fluid that is mixed with sperm to facilitate its passage through urethra during ejaculation.

Urethra
Channel passing through prostate gland down center of penis. Permits exit of sperm and seminal fluid during ejaculation; also permits exit of urine from bladder during urination.

Seminal vesicle
Cystic structure between bladder and rectum stores sperm for ejaculation.

Ejaculatory duct
Opening of seminal vesicle into urethra through which sperm passes during ejaculation.

Vas deferens
Channel that carries sperm from testicle to seminal vesicle for storage.

Testicle
One of two identical male sex organs. Produces sperm for storage until ejaculation. Also secretes hormone called testosterone into blood to stimulate genital and hair development as well as voice change during adolescence. Testicles held inside fleshy sac called scrotum.

Pituitary gland
Master gland of endocrine system controlled by adjoining brain section called hypothalamus. Releases hormones into blood that stimulate other endocrine glands such as adrenal glands and testicles to release their hormones.

Adrenal gland
One of two identical endocrine glands located above kidneys. Responds to strong emotion by releasing hormone called adrenalin into blood to speed heart rate and breathing, and prepare muscles for action. Also releases small amount of male sex hormone.

TROUBLESHOOTING GUIDE

PROBLEM	PROCEDURE
FEMALE	
Pregnancy; anxiousness	Ensure safe pregnancy (p. 87)
	Consult a physician if breathlessness during first trimester or at rest, nausea and vomiting after first trimester, vaginal bleeding at any time, a weight gain of more than 4 pounds in one week, or a weight loss of more than 2 pounds in one week
Puberty; anxiousness	Monitor adolescent sexual development (p. 90) and consult a physician about any suspected physical or emotional problem
Vaginal discharge	Maintain personal hygiene (p. 91) and consult a physician
	If recommended, choose alternative contraception method (p. 87)
Vaginal odor	Maintain personal hygiene (p. 91) and consult a physician
	If recommended, choose alternative contraception method (p. 87)
Genital rash, sore, blister or pimple	Maintain personal hygiene (p. 91) and consult a physician
Genital irritation: swelling, itching, burning, tenderness or soreness	Maintain personal hygiene (p. 91) and consult a physician
	If recommended, choose alternative contraception method (p. 87)
Unexpected vaginal bleeding	Seek emergency help ✚ if bleeding severe or occurs during pregnancy
	Consult a physician; if recommended, choose alternative contraception method (p. 87)
Menstrual abnormality: period irregular, absent, or suddenly or increasing painful or heavy	Consult a physician; if recommended, choose alternative contraception method (p. 87)
Breast abnormality: lump, swelling, tenderness or pain; discharge or bleeding from nipple	Consult a physician and perform regular breast self-examination (p. 88)
Urination painful, burning	Maintain personal hygiene (p. 91) and consult a physician
	If necessary, treat urinary tract infection (p. 83)
MALE	
Puberty; anxiousness	Monitor adolescent sexual development (p. 90) and consult a physician about any suspected physical or emotional problem
Discharge from urethra	Maintain personal hygiene (p. 91) and consult a physician
Blood in semen	Consult a physician
Testicle abnormality: feeling of heaviness, tenderness or pain; unusual swelling or lumpiness; bleeding	Consult a physician and perform regular testicle self-examination (p. 89)
Genital odor	Maintain personal hygiene (p. 91)
Genital rash, sore, blister or pimple	Maintain personal hygiene (p. 91) and consult a physician
Genital irritation: swelling, itching, burning, tenderness or soreness	Maintain personal hygiene (p. 91) and consult a physician
Urination painful, burning	Maintain personal hygiene (p. 91) and consult a physician
	If necessary, treat urinary tract infection (p. 83)
Urination frequent or difficult	Reduce consumption of liquids—especially beverages of alcohol and caffeine
	Watch for and treat any secondary problem
	Consult a physician if urination interrupts daily routines or sleeping habits; if necessary, manage prostate gland disorder (p. 90)
Urinary control loss	Consult a physician; if necessary, manage prostate gland disorder (p. 90)
Urination inability	Consult a physician if inability to urinate lasts more than 24 hours; if necessary, manage prostate gland disorder (p. 90)
Urine discolored: dark or red	Consult a physician; if necessary, manage prostate gland disorder (p. 90)

✚ **Medical emergency**

CHOOSING A CONTRACEPTIVE METHOD

Using contraceptive devices. A variety of methods are available to undertake effective family planning and prevent unwanted pregnancy; in addition, the proper use of a condom can significantly reduce the risk of contracting a sexually-transmitted disease. Consult a physician to discuss your contraceptive options. If you choose natural contraception using a technique such as the rythm method, ensure that the physician explains carefully how to estimate your safe period for sexual activity. If you choose artificial contraception, evaluate the contraceptive devices available *(right)*, selecting one that you are comfortable using. To use any contraceptive device, carefully follow the physician's directions, as well as any instructions provided by the manufacturer. Be alert to the possible side effects of using a contraceptive device: genital irritation; vaginal discharge or odor; unexpected bleeding or a menstrual abnormality. If you suspect that a contraceptive device is responsible for a problem, discontinue your use of it and consult a physician. Then, if necessary, choose an alternative contraceptive method.

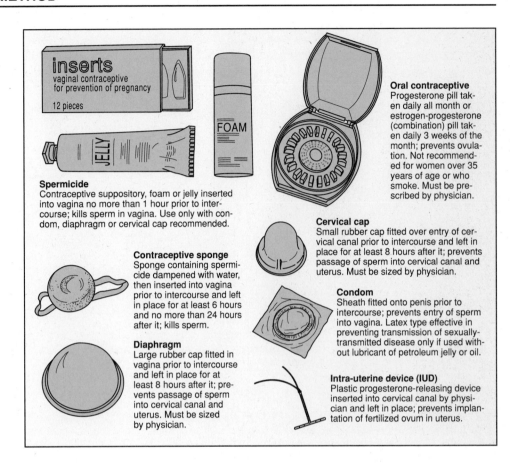

Spermicide
Contraceptive suppository, foam or jelly inserted into vagina no more than 1 hour prior to intercourse; kills sperm in vagina. Use only with condom, diaphragm or cervical cap recommended.

Contraceptive sponge
Sponge containing spermicide dampened with water, then inserted into vagina prior to intercourse and left in place for at least 6 hours and no more than 24 hours after it; kills sperm.

Diaphragm
Large rubber cap fitted in vagina prior to intercourse and left in place for at least 8 hours after it; prevents passage of sperm into cervical canal and uterus. Must be sized by physician.

Oral contraceptive
Progesterone pill taken daily all month or estrogen-progesterone (combination) pill taken daily 3 weeks of the month; prevents ovulation. Not recommended for women over 35 years of age or who smoke. Must be prescribed by physician.

Cervical cap
Small rubber cap fitted over entry of cervical canal prior to intercourse and left in place for at least 8 hours after it; prevents passage of sperm into cervical canal and uterus. Must be sized by physician.

Condom
Sheath fitted onto penis prior to intercourse; prevents entry of sperm into vagina. Latex type effective in preventing transmission of sexually-transmitted disease only if used without lubricant of petroleum jelly or oil.

Intra-uterine device (IUD)
Plastic progesterone-releasing device inserted into cervical canal by physician and left in place; prevents implantation of fertilized ovum in uterus.

MANAGING PREGNANCY

Ensuring a safe pregnancy. Most women carry a child from conception through delivery without major problems. However, pregnancy can be a time of anxiety, uncertainty and fear—about a possible miscarriage or birth defect, the experience of labor and childbirth, or the many unknown demands of a new baby. Adequate prenatal care is essential; ask your physician to recommend an obstetrician and a pediatrician, and find out about the prenatal services available in your community.

• Avoid morning sickness by preventing hunger. Eat crackers or dry toast before leaving bed; have light snacks during the day.

• Eat a regular, well-balanced diet. Avoid anemia by eating foods rich in iron such as liver, whole-grain or enriched bread, dried fruit and green vegetables.

• Do not smoke or drink alcohol or coffee; toxins pass easily across the placental barrier and can cause damage to a fetus.

• Prevent varicose veins by wearing comfortable clothing that fits loosely around the waist and legs; sit with the feet elevated as often and as long as possible.

• To minimize heartburn eat small, frequent meals; sleep propped up in bed with extra pillows.

Be alert to the warning signs of a serious problem during a pregnancy and consult a physician immediately about any of the following symptoms: breathlessness during the first trimester or at rest; nausea and vomiting after the first trimester; vaginal bleeding at any time; a weight gain of more than 4 pounds in one week; or, a weight loss of more than 2 pounds in one week.

Refer to the guidelines presented below to help you manage a comfortable and safe pregnancy:

• Do not use a nonprescription medication without the approval of your physician; carefully follow directions for any needed medication, observing any warnings about its use during pregnancy.

• To help relieve ankle swelling, avoid standing for prolonged periods of time. Sit with the feet elevated as often and as long as possible. Wear properly-fitting footwear with flat heels.

• Maintain a regular program of moderate physical exercise; activities such as walking or swimming, for example, can help improve fitness and enhance physical condition. Avoid strenuous physical exercise, however; do not use a sauna, a steam bath, a hot tub or a whirlpool.

• Avoid contact with anyone suffering an infectious disease such as German measles (rubella) that can seriously damage a fetus.

PERFORMING A BREAST SELF-EXAMINATION

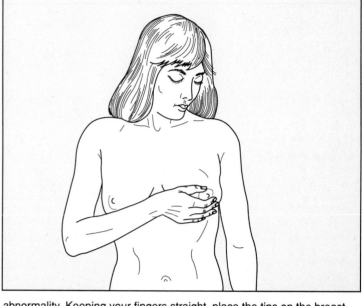

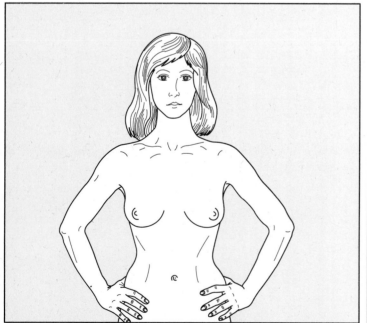

1 **Feeling for abnormalities while standing.** Closely examine the breasts on the same day every month to help you detect any abnormality that may be an early warning sign of cancer or another disorder. Examine the breasts 7 to 10 days following menstruation; if you no longer menstruate, on a set day of the month. Start by feeling for abnormalities while standing in the shower; warm, soapy water helps the fingers glide smoothly over the breast and detect any change in it. Examine each breast in turn, resting the arm on the same side of the body on your head and using the opposite hand to feel for any abnormality. Keeping your fingers straight, place the tips on the breast just above the nipple and press gently *(above, left)*, feeling for any lump or thickening of the skin, or any tenderness or pain. Continue to feel the breast for abnormalities the same way, repositioning your fingertips at points across it, then at points under and along the sides of it. After feeling the breast, use the thumb and forefinger of your hand to gently squeeze the nipple *(above, right)*, checking for discharge or any tenderness or pain; unless you are lactating, there should be no discharge.

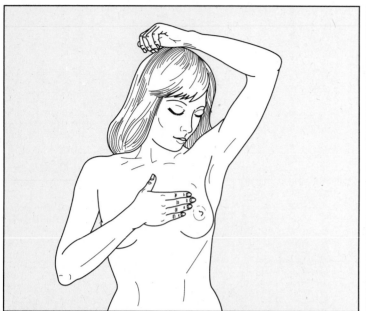

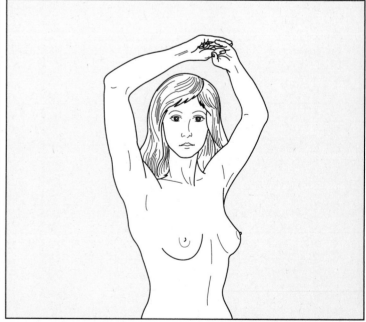

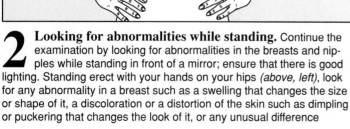

2 **Looking for abnormalities while standing.** Continue the examination by looking for abnormalities in the breasts and nipples while standing in front of a mirror; ensure that there is good lighting. Standing erect with your hands on your hips *(above, left)*, look for any abnormality in a breast such as a swelling that changes the size or shape of it, a discoloration or a distortion of the skin such as dimpling or puckering that changes the look of it, or any unusual difference between the two breasts. Also look for any abnormality in a nipple such as an excessive outward or upward thrust, or any sign of bleeding or weeping. Then, stand erect with your arms above your head and repeat the inspection, examining the breasts and nipples in turn from the front, then from each side *(above, right)*. Pay especially close attention to the undersides of the breasts and the armpits.

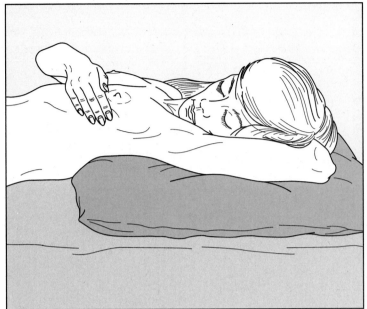

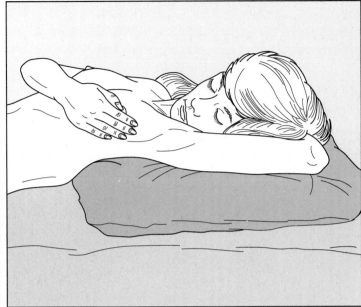

3 **Feeling for abnormalities while lying down.** Finish the examination by feeling for abnormalities in the breasts while lying down, distributing the breast tissue evenly across the chest. Examine each breast in turn, lying with a pillow under the shoulder on the same side of the body. Resting the arm on the same side of the body as the breast above your head, use the opposite hand to feel for abnormalities. Keeping your fingers straight, place the tips on the breast just above the nipple and press gently, feeling for any lump or thickening of the skin, or any tenderness or pain. Continue to feel the breast for abnormalities the same way, repositioning your fingertips at points across it, then at points under *(above, left)* and along the sides of it *(above, right)*. Pay especially close attention to the armpits. Consult a physician about any abnormality detected during a self-examination.

PERFORMING A TESTICLE SELF-EXAMINATION

Detecting a testicle disorder. Research done by the American Cancer Society indicates that testicular cancer is the most common form of cancer that affects men between the ages of 18 and 35. Any male between 15 and 40 years of age at risk for the development of testicular cancer should perform a regular testicle self-examination *(step right)* to help detect the early warning signs of possible cancer or other disorder of the testicles. When a tumor is detected early and treated promptly, the chances of a complete cure—whether by radiation therapy or surgery—are excellent.

Be alert to an unusual problem that may indicate a possible disorder of the testicles, particularly if a symptom is persistent or recurs. Consult a physician if you notice any of the following:

• heaviness of the testicles

• tenderness or pain in the testicles

• unusual hardness of the testicles

• swelling or bleeding of the testicles

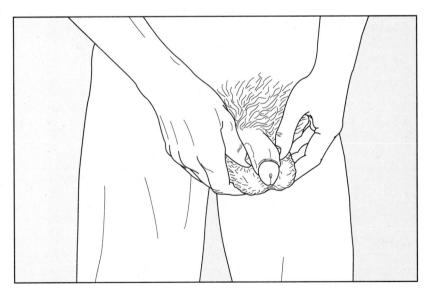

Feeling the testicles for abnormalities. Closely examine the testicles once each month after taking a warm bath or shower—while the genital skin and muscles are warm and relaxed. Examine one testicle at a time, gently feeling the scrotum to locate it; if you cannot find a testicle or it is located high up in the scrotum, suspect that it has not descended properly and consult a physician. To examine the testicle, hold it between your hands, placing your thumbs on top of it and your fingers under it *(above)*; if necessary, separate your legs for better access to it. Gently roll the testicle between your thumbs and fingers to feel for any abnormality such as a lump or hard spot, or any pain. Consult a physician about any abnormality detected—including any unusual difference between the testicles.

MANAGING A PROSTATE GLAND DISORDER

Detecting the early warning signs of a prostate disorder. Disorders of the prostate gland are especially common in men over 50 years of age; any male over 40 years of age should request a prostate examination as part of an annual medical checkup. While the symptoms of a prostate gland disorder vary according to the type of disorder, any prostate gland disorder is characterized by marked changes in urinary habits. Use the information below to familiarize yourself with the symptoms of two common prostate disorders: prostatitis and prostate enlargement. Report any suspected disorder to a physician as soon as possible:

• **Prostatitis.** Prostatitis is inflammation of the prostate gland due to a bacterial infection—often affecting men under the age of 40. Prostatitis can produce the following urinary symptoms: a feeling of heaviness or painful swelling between the scrotum and the anus; a frequent, sudden and urgent need to urinate; painful, burning urination or pain in the lower abdomen during urination; discolored urine; and a high fever. Consult a physician about a suspected case of prostatitis; if requested, collect a urine sample (page 83) to bring to the consultation. To assist in making a diagnosis, the physician may do a rectal examination, inserting a finger through the anus into the rectum to feel for any abnormality of the prostate gland. If prostatitis is diagnosed, the physician may prescribe antibiotics. To cure prostatitis effectively, carefully follow the physician's directions to use any medication; use the amount specified at the prescribed times and report any side effect to the physician. Get plenty of rest and drink lots of fluids, avoiding any consumption of alcohol. To relieve any discomfort, sit in a warm bath.

• **Prostate enlargement.** Enlargement of the prostate gland due to hormonal changes that result from aging is a common problem of men over the age of 50. An enlarged prostate gland can produce the following symptoms: frequent need to urinate, especially during the night; difficult urination that is hard to start, produces a hesitant stream of urine, and ends with prolonged dribbling along with the feeling of a still-full bladder; and prolonged, painful erections. Consult a physician about a suspected case of prostate enlargement; if requested, collect a urine sample (page 83) to bring to the consultation. To assist in making a diagnosis, the physician may do a rectal examination, inserting a finger through the anus into the rectum to feel for any abnormality of the prostate gland. If a prostate enlargement is diagnosed, surgery may be recommended. To manage a condition of prostate enlargement that does not require surgery, avoid alcohol consumption and keep the bladder as empty as possible, urinating frequently. To relieve any discomfort and help ease difficult urination, sit in a warm bath.

MANAGING PUBERTY

Monitoring adolescent development.

Puberty is the period of adolescence during which a young boy or girl enters manhood or womanhood, attaining the physical ability to reproduce. The sex hormones testosterone, estrogen, and progesterone—all present to some degree in males and females—cause the changes that accompany puberty. In males, the testicles produce testosterone, the key hormone for stimulating sexual development of a boy. In females, the ovaries produce estrogen and progesterone, the key hormones responsible for stimulating sexual development of a girl.

The onset and duration of puberty are governed by heredity and the general health of an adolescent. The sexual development of a boy usually follows the pattern of the father; the sexual development of a girl usually follows the pattern of the mother. However, for an adolescent who suffers a chronic physical disorder, puberty can be delayed. Because of wide variations in adolescent sexual development patterns, an early- or late-bloomer is often subjected to unwanted attention from peers.

Parents should be alert to any emotional difficulty accompanying the sexual development of an adolescent; help to alleviate any distress by providing empathetic support, assuring that any differences are only temporary and that growth to maturity is usually completed by age 18. Use the chart at right to help monitor the sexual development of an adolescent; do not hesitate to consult a physician if an adolescent's sexual development is unusually rapid or slow, or an adolescent is having emotional difficulty during puberty.

PHYSICAL CHANGE OF FEMALE	AVERAGE AGE
Growth rate increase	10 to 16 years of age; consult a physician if no growth by 15 years of age
Breast development	10 to 14 years of age; consult a physician if no breast development by 16 years of age
Body hair emergence	10 to 14 years of age for pubic hair and 12 to 16 years of age for underarm hair; amount varies according to heredity
Menstruation	11 to 17 years of age, often irregularly; consult a physician if menstruation begins before 10 years of age or has not begun by 17 years of age

PHYSICAL CHANGE OF MALE	AVERAGE AGE
Growth rate increase	12 to 18 years of age; consult a physician if no growth by 15 years of age
Genital enlargement	11 to 17 years of age for testicle growth and 12 to 16 years of age for penis growth; consult a physician if no genital development by 16 years of age
Body hair emergence	11 to 16 years of age for pubic hair and 13 to 18 years of age for underarm hair; amount varies according to heredity
Voice change	13 to 14 years of age for enlargement of voicebox and 14 to 17 years of age for deepening of voice

MAINTAINING PERSONAL HYGIENE

Maintaining genital hygiene. Because of their warmth and moisture, the genitals are prone to many minor irritations and infections. Proper genital hygiene, however, can help prevent the onset of a problem; in particular, teach young children and maturing adolescents about the importance of genital hygiene. In general, any

• Males and females should avoid wearing undergarments of synthetic fibers that can restrict air circulation and encourage bacterial infections. Wear undergarments of a natural fiber such as cotton.

• Males and females should clean the genitals daily. Use a soft, clean facecloth to wash the genitals thoroughly with an unscented soap and water; an uncircumcised male should also draw back the foreskin to clean under it. Then, rinse the area well with fresh water and dry it thoroughly with a clean towel.

• A female should avoid using a vaginal deodorant spray unless recommended by a physician; many products contain substances that can cause irritation. To use a deodorant spray, carefully follow

sore, swelling, rash, itching or pain of the genital area should be reported to a physician as soon as possible. Avoid using a nonprescription medication to relieve any genital irritation unless recommended by your physician. Refer to the guidelines below to help you maintain proper hygiene:

the manufacturer's directions to apply it; avoid spraying any product directly into the vagina. Discontinue the use of a product if it causes a vaginal irritation.

• A female should avoid douching, especially if she has a vaginal infection. Douching can wash away the mucous lining of the cervix that prevents infectious organisms from entering the uterine cavity. Douching can also disturb the chemical balance of the vagina.

• A female should avoid using scented tampons or hygienic pads to reduce odor during menstruation; many products contain substances that can cause irritation. Wash the genital area thoroughly with soap and water daily; change tampons or pads frequently.

Maintaining sexual hygiene. A sexually-transmitted disease (STD) is a genital or urinary disorder acquired through sexual contact with an infected person. While STDs are not problems for most individuals, recent attention to the spread of Acquired Immune Deficiency Syndrome (AIDS) has convinced more people of the importance of sexually hygienic practices.

While medical research has yielded effective treatments for many disorders, the best cure remains prevention. The proper use of a condom, for example, can minimize the risk of acquiring an infection from a sexual partner. Proper genital hygiene (*step above*) before and after sexual contact can also prevent many minor irritations of the genital area. As an added precaution, a sexually active person should request tests for STDs as part of an annual medical checkup.

In general, any sore, swelling, rash, itching or pain of the genital area should be reported to a physician as soon as possible; or, a person with a suspected STD may wish to go to a clinic that specializes in STDs. Use the chart at right to help familiarize yourself with the symptoms and procedures for managing a suspected STD.

DISORDER	SYMPTOMS AND TREATMENT
Gonorrhea	In female, often no symptoms; may cause urethral discharge and burning, frequent urination. In male, causes urethral discharge and burning, frequent urination. Stop sexual activity and consult physician for swab test. Use any prescription antibiotics exactly as prescribed and report for any follow-up tests. Inform sexual partner of positive diagnosis and remain abstinent until physician confirms cure of infection.
Chlamydia (non-specific urethral infection)	Often no symptoms; may cause slight urethral discharge and tingling during urination. Stop sexual activity and consult physician for swab test. Use any prescription antibiotics exactly as prescribed and report for any follow-up tests. Inform sexual partner of positive diagnosis and remain abstinent until physician confirms cure of infection.
Syphilis	In primary stage, causes small painless, ulcer-like sore on penis or on vulva or vagina; may be accompanied by swollen lymph glands (*page 62*). In secondary stage, causes extensive rash, often on palms of hands and soles of feet; may be accompanied by fever. Stop sexual activity and consult physician for blood test. Use any prescription antibiotics exactly as prescribed and report for any follow-up tests. Inform sexual partner of positive diagnosis and remain abstinent until physician confirms cure of infection.
Genital herpes	Causes recurring eruptions of tiny, painful blisters that break and form crusts on genitals and possibly thighs or buttocks; may be accompanied by swollen lymph glands (*page 62*), fever and burning, frequent urination. Stop sexual activity and consult physician for examination. Use any prescription antiviral medication exactly as prescribed. Inform sexual partner of positive diagnosis, remain abstinent during any recurrence, and use condom.
Pubic lice (crabs)	Causes intense itching of genital area, especially in pubic hair. Stop sexual activity and consult physician for examination. Use any prescription lotion or ointment exactly as prescribed and report for any follow-up tests; thoroughly launder all linens and clothing in hot water. Inform sexual partner of positive diagnosis and remain abstinent until physician confirms cure of problem.
Venereal warts	Causes eruption of tiny, painless, cauliflower-like growths on penis or vulva, or on anus. Stop sexual activity and consult physician for examination; minor surgery to remove warts may be recommended. For contagious warts, inform sexual partner of positive diagnosis and remain abstinent until physician confirms cure of problem.

EYES AND EARS

Your eyes and ears are the organs that provide you with the ability to see and hear—the two most important senses by which you understand and respond to the environment around you. The diagrams on page 93 illustrate the complex and delicate structures that comprise the eye and the ear. In the eye, the cornea and iris work to let light pass through the pupil where it is focused and projected by the lens onto the retina; the retina transmits the light as an electrical impulse along the optic nerve to the brain. The eye is protected and cleaned by the eyelids, eyelashes, and lacrimal (tear) glands and ducts. In the ear, sound waves entering the outer ear and ear canal strike and vibrate the ear drum and bones of the middle ear, then the fluid-filled cochlea of the inner ear; the cochlea transmits the vibration as an electrical impulse along the auditory nerve to the brain. The inner ear also houses the semi-circular canals, the body's organs of balance.

Although disorders of the eyes and ears are not common household medical problems, the importance and delicacy of these sense organs means any problem that does arise should be attended to by a physician, especially if it is persistent or recurs. The Troubleshooting Guide *(page 94)* puts procedures for common eye and ear problems at your fingertips and refers you to pages 95 to 99 for more detailed information. Familiarize yourself with the techniques for treating a black eye *(page 95)*, removing a particle from an eye *(page 96)* and dislodging an object from an ear *(page 99)*.

For an injury to an eye from a chemical splash, a laceration or an embedded object, seek emergency help; first, however, take the first-aid steps necessary to flush a chemical from the eye *(page 95)* or stabilize an object embedded in the eye *(page 96)* and prevent eye movement *(page 96)*, minimizing further damage to the eye. For techniques on handling a life-threatening emergency such as a head injury that affects the eyes or ears, consult the Emergency Guide *(page 8)*. For techniques on caring for a family member who is ill or recuperating from an illness, consult the Equipment & Techniques chapter *(page 110)*.

The list of health tips at right covers basic guidelines for preventing eye and ear problems. Always wear the proper safety equipment to undertake physical work or a sport that might injure the eyes or damage the hearing. An annual hearing test and eye examination are excellent preventive measures, especially if there is a family history of hearing difficulties or eye problems such as glaucoma. If you must cope with an eye or ear problem at home, do not hesitate to call for help; medical professionals can answer questions about symptoms and treatments. Post the telephone numbers for your physician, local hospital emergency room, ambulance and pharmacy near the telephone; in most regions, dial 911 in the event of a life-threatening emergency. Keep handy the telephone number of an ear, nose and throat specialist and an opthalmologist recommended by your physician.

HEALTH TIPS

1. Never insert any object into the ear canal. In particular, educate a small child about the danger of inserting small toys such as sticks and beads into the ear canal.

2. Use a cotton swab to clean wax from the ear only if the wax is visible at the outer edge of the ear canal or in the folds of the outer ear. Never insert a cotton swab into the ear canal to clean out wax; wax protects the ear from infection and removing it risks damaging the ear.

3. If you suspect that minor hearing difficulty may be due to excess wax in the ear, consult a physician to examine the ear and, if necessary, to remove the wax.

4. Prevent hearing damage by using hearing protection *(page 98)* to protect the ears from high-intensity noise when working with power tools such as routers, sanders and power saws.

5. To help prevent the development of a major ear problem, talk to your physician about having an annual hearing test, especially if there is a family history of hearing difficulties.

6. To help prevent the development of a major eye problem, have an eye examination annually. Be aware of any family history of eye problems such as glaucoma; an adult at risk should have an annual visual field test.

7. Consult a physician immediately about any potentially-serious eye or ear symptom such as pain, bleeding or any deterioration of sight or hearing.

8. Avoid touching or rubbing the eyes, especially if the hands are not clean. Never touch the cornea or pupil of an eye.

9. Prevent eye damage by using eye protection *(page 98)* to shield the eyes from flying particles or chemical splashes when working. Use protective goggles to swim in chlorinated water or for any activity such as a racquet sport in which there is a risk of eye injury.

10. To prevent eye strain and fatigue, always work with proper lighting. Whenever the eyes begin to tire, stop and rest.

11. Never look directly at the sun or a bright light source. To protect your eyes from sunlight, consult your physician or an opthalmologist for proper sunglasses; avoid buying inexpensive glasses that provide poor eye protection.

12. If you wear contact lenses, use only the cleaning solution and lubricant prescribed for them exactly as prescribed; consult your opthalmologist about any problem with the contact lenses. Never share contact lenses with others.

13. Avoid using nonprescription drops for the eyes or ears unless recommended by your physician. Some preparations may irritate or injure the eyes or ears if used incorrectly.

14. Carefully follow the physician's directions to use any prescription medication for an eye or ear ailment; use only the amount specified at only the prescribed times and report any side effect to the physician.

EYE

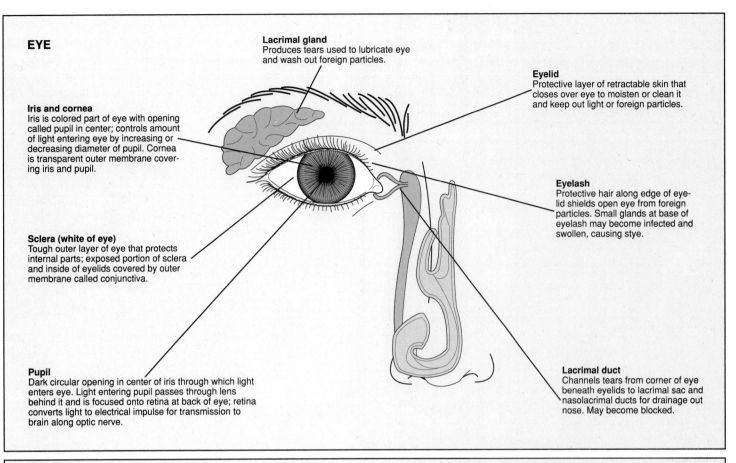

Lacrimal gland
Produces tears used to lubricate eye and wash out foreign particles.

Eyelid
Protective layer of retractable skin that closes over eye to moisten or clean it and keep out light or foreign particles.

Iris and cornea
Iris is colored part of eye with opening called pupil in center; controls amount of light entering eye by increasing or decreasing diameter of pupil. Cornea is transparent outer membrane covering iris and pupil.

Eyelash
Protective hair along edge of eyelid shields open eye from foreign particles. Small glands at base of eyelash may become infected and swollen, causing stye.

Sclera (white of eye)
Tough outer layer of eye that protects internal parts; exposed portion of sclera and inside of eyelids covered by outer membrane called conjunctiva.

Pupil
Dark circular opening in center of iris through which light enters eye. Light entering pupil passes through lens behind it and is focused onto retina at back of eye; retina converts light to electrical impulse for transmission to brain along optic nerve.

Lacrimal duct
Channels tears from corner of eye beneath eyelids to lacrimal sac and nasolacrimal ducts for drainage out nose. May become blocked.

EAR

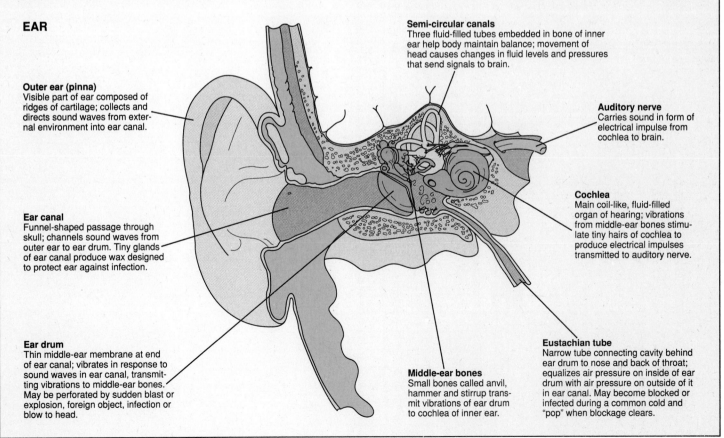

Semi-circular canals
Three fluid-filled tubes embedded in bone of inner ear help body maintain balance; movement of head causes changes in fluid levels and pressures that send signals to brain.

Outer ear (pinna)
Visible part of ear composed of ridges of cartilage; collects and directs sound waves from external environment into ear canal.

Auditory nerve
Carries sound in form of electrical impulse from cochlea to brain.

Ear canal
Funnel-shaped passage through skull; channels sound waves from outer ear to ear drum. Tiny glands of ear canal produce wax designed to protect ear against infection.

Cochlea
Main coil-like, fluid-filled organ of hearing; vibrations from middle-ear bones stimulate tiny hairs of cochlea to produce electrical impulses transmitted to auditory nerve.

Ear drum
Thin middle-ear membrane at end of ear canal; vibrates in response to sound waves in ear canal, transmitting vibrations to middle-ear bones. May be perforated by sudden blast or explosion, foreign object, infection or blow to head.

Middle-ear bones
Small bones called anvil, hammer and stirrup transmit vibrations of ear drum to cochlea of inner ear.

Eustachian tube
Narrow tube connecting cavity behind ear drum to nose and back of throat; equalizes air pressure on inside of ear drum with air pressure on outside of it in ear canal. May become blocked or infected during a common cold and "pop" when blockage clears.

TROUBLESHOOTING GUIDE

PROBLEM	PROCEDURE
EYE	
Blow to face or head near eye	Seek emergency help ✚ if injury severe; if necessary, use emergency first aid *(p. 8)*
	Prevent a black eye *(p. 95)*
	Watch for and treat any secondary problem
	Consult a physician if visual impairment follows injury, pain or swelling lasts more than 3 days, or discoloration or tenderness lasts more than 3 weeks
Wound to eye	Prevent eye movement *(p. 97)*, then seek emergency help ✚
Chemical in eye	Flush chemical from eye *(p. 95)* and prevent eye movement *(p. 97)*, then seek emergency help ✚
Particle in eye	Do not rub eye; do not attempt to remove particle if on cornea, embedded or adhered
	Remove particle from eye *(p. 96)* and prevent eye movement *(p. 97)*, then seek emergency help ✚
Object embedded in eye	Do not attempt to remove object from eye
	Stabilize embedded object *(p. 97)*, then seek emergency help ✚
Stye suspected: painful, red swelling of eyelid	Administer heat treatment *(p. 119)* for 10 minutes every 2 to 3 hours
	Consult a physician if stye does not discharge after 3 days
Conjunctivitis suspected: white of eye red and sticky; feeling of gritty irritation in eye	Rest eye and avoid exposure to airborne irritants; do not patch or cover eye
	Administer heat treatment *(p. 119)* for 10 minutes every 2 to 3 hours
	Consult a physician if irritation lasts more than 3 days or episodes of irritation recur
Pain, irritation in eyeball	Seek emergency help ✚ if pain or irritation sudden and severe
	Watch for and treat any secondary problem
	Consult a physician if irritation lasts more than 3 days or episodes of irritation recur
Visual impairment: blurred vision; cloudy vision; double-image vision; tunnel vision; black dots or filaments in field of vision; visual field partly obscured	Seek emergency help ✚ if impairment sudden and severe
	Watch for and treat any secondary problem
	Consult a physician if impairment lasts more than 3 days or episodes of impairment recur
Loss of vision	Seek emergency help ✚
EAR	
Blow to face or head near ear	Seek emergency help ✚ if injury severe; if necessary, use emergency first aid *(p. 8)*
	Watch for and treat any secondary problem
	Consult a physician if earache or hearing impairment follows injury
Wound to outer ear	Seek emergency help ✚ if bleeding severe or wound deep or gaping
	Stop any bleeding and bandage ear *(p. 99)*
	Consult a physician for tetanus treatment if wound caused by rusty or dirty object
	Watch for and treat any secondary problem
Object in ear	Seek emergency help ✚ if there is severe pain or bleeding, or discharge from ear canal
	Dislodge object from ear *(p. 99)*
	Watch for and treat any secondary problem
Wax in ear	Use cotton swab to clean only outer edge of ear canal and folds of outer ear; do not insert cotton swab into ear canal
	Consult a physician to examine ear and, if necessary, remove ear wax
Earache	Seek emergency help ✚ if there is severe pain or bleeding, or discharge from ear canal
	Rest; use nonprescription pain-reliever *(p. 121)*
	Watch for and treat any secondary problem
	Consult a physician if earache lasts more than 12 hours
Bleeding or discharge from ear canal	Seek emergency help ✚
Hearing impairment: buzzing, ringing, humming or tinkling sounds; blockage	Seek emergency help ✚ if impairment sudden and severe
	Watch for and treat any secondary problem
	Consult a physician if impairment worsens or episodes of impairment recur
Loss of hearing	Seek emergency help ✚

✚ **Medical emergency**

PREVENTING A BLACK EYE

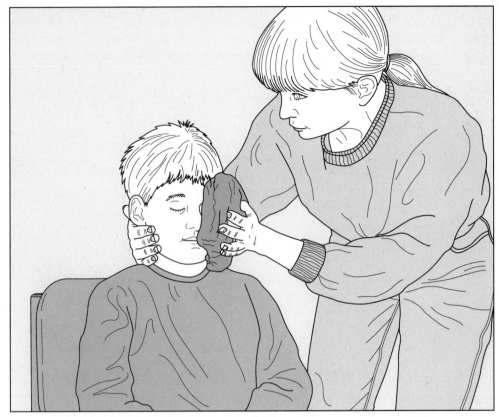

Applying a cold compress. If a blow to the head or face injures the eye, prevent eye movement *(page 97)* and seek medical help immediately. Otherwise, to relieve pain or swelling and minimize the bruising that can cause a black eye, administer cold treatments for 48 hours, then heat treatments. Lie or sit in a comfortable position and close the eyes. For a cold treatment, apply an ice pack or a plastic bag of ice cubes wrapped in a towel *(left)* for 15 to 20 minutes. For a heat treatment, apply a clean facecloth soaked in hot—not scalding—water the same way. Consult a physician if any impairment of vision, pain or swelling lasts more than 3 days, or discoloration or tenderness lasts more than 3 weeks.

CLEARING A CHEMICAL FROM THE EYE

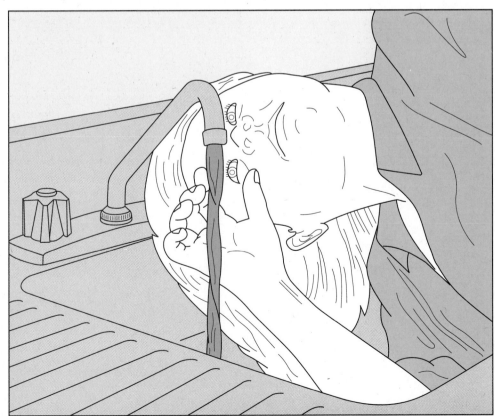

Flushing a chemical from the eye. **Caution:** Do not rub the eye. Holding the eyelids of the injured eye apart with your fingers, position it under a gentle flow of cool water from a faucet *(left)* or pitcher; tilt the head to one side to keep the chemical from washing into the uninjured eye. If you are outdoors, flush the injured eye the same way using a flow of water from a garden hose. **Caution:** Remove any nozzle from the garden hose to prevent an eye injury from a strong jet of water. Do not allow a child to flush an injured eye on his own; hold his head with one hand and use the other hand to flush the injured eye for him. Flush the injured eye for 15 to 30 minutes, then prevent eye movement *(page 97)* and seek medical help immediately.

CLEARING A PARTICLE FROM THE EYE

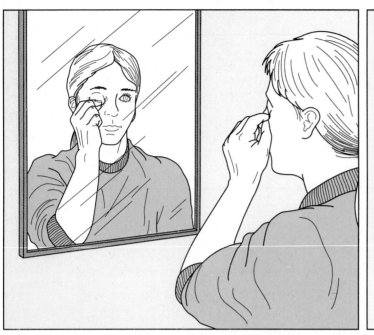

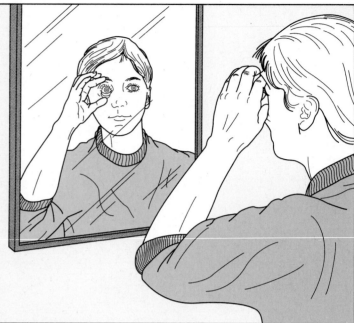

1 **Removing a particle from the white of the eye. Caution:** Do not rub the eye. First, try to remove the particle by making the eye water. Gently grasp the lashes of the upper eyelid to pull it down over the lower eyelid *(above, left)*. If you cannot wash out the particle, locate it to remove it. Facing a mirror, use the forefinger and thumb of one hand to hold open the injured eye, then inspect the surface of it for the particle *(above, right)*; if necessary, slowly rotate the eye to help expose the particle. **Caution:** If a particle is on the cornea or appears to be adhered or embedded, do not remove it; prevent any eye movement *(page 97)* and seek medical help immediately. If you cannot see the particle on the surface of the eye, check for it under the eyelids *(step 2)*. Otherwise, remove the particle from the white of the eye using the twisted end of a tissue moistened with water.

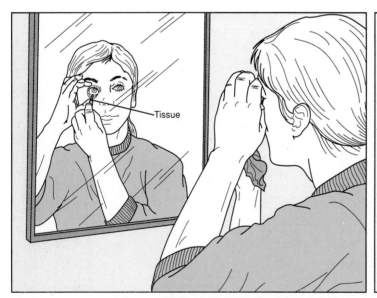

Tissue

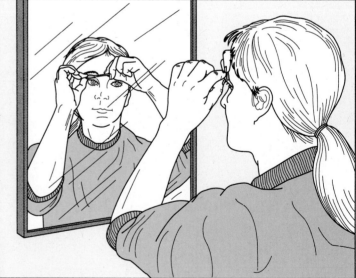

2 **Removing a particle from under an eyelid.** To check for a particle under the lower eyelid, hold the eye open and gently push the lower lid down. Remove the particle from the inside of the lid by gently dabbing it using the twisted end of a tissue moistened with water *(above, left)*. To check for a particle under the upper eyelid, hold a clean cotton swab against the bottom edge of it, then gently grasp the lashes to fold the lid back against the cotton swab *(above, right)*. Remove the particle from the underside of the lid by having a helper gently dab it using the twisted end of a tissue moistened with water. If you cannot locate the particle on the surface of the eye or under an eyelid, flush the eye *(page 95)* for several minutes. If the problem persists, prevent any eye movement *(page 97)* and seek medical help immediately.

PREVENTING EYE MOVEMENT

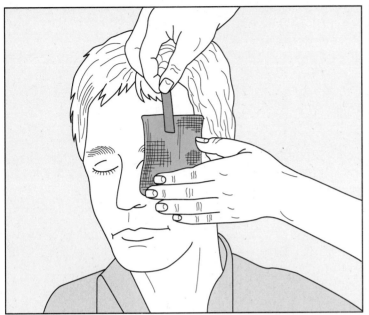
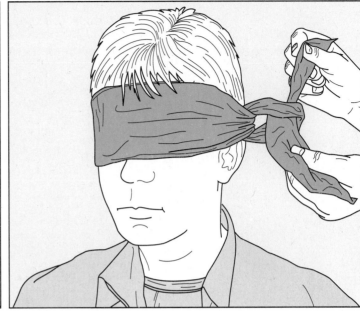

Applying eye dressings. To protect an injured eye from further damage until it can be attended to by a physician, prevent eye movement by covering both eyes with dressings. Have the
victim close his eyes and sit or lie still; do not allow him to open or touch his eyes. Gently place
a sterile gauze dressing over the injured eye. Without exerting pressure on the eye, secure the
dressing using adhesive tape *(above, left)*. Repeat the procedure on the other eye. Then, bandage the dressings in place using a folded triangular bandage or a scarf. Position the bandage
over the eyes and around the victim's head, tying it snugly at the side of the head *(above, right)*.
Seek medical help immediately.

STABILIZING AN OBJECT EMBEDDED IN THE EYE

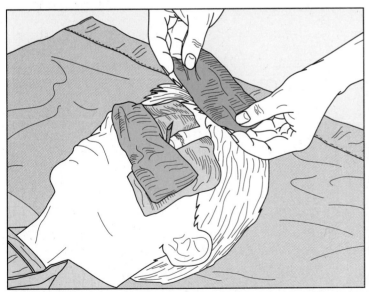
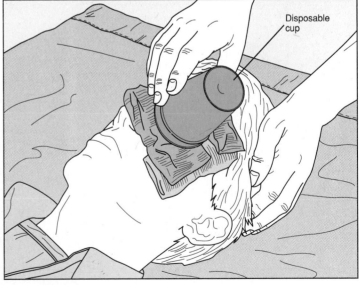

Disposable cup

1 Making a covering. Caution: Do not attempt to pull out an object embedded in an eye;
seek medical help immediately. If the object protrudes from the eye, protect the eye from
further injury by securing a covering over the object to stabilize it. Have the victim sit or lie
still; do not allow him to touch his eyes. To make a covering, build up a ring of gauze dressings
around the base of the object *(above, left)*, making sure that you apply no pressure on the
embedded object or the eye. Then, position a disposable cup or cone upside down over the
object, resting it gently on the ring of dressings *(above, right)*. Secure the covering *(step 2)*.

STABILIZING AN OBJECT EMBEDDED IN THE EYE (continued)

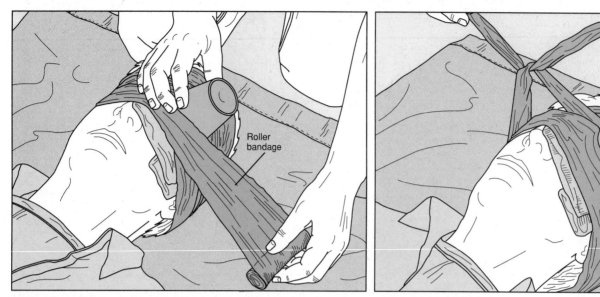

Roller
bandage

2 **Securing the covering.** Secure the covering using a gauze roller bandage; if necessary, have a helper hold the covering steady while you secure it. Starting at the side of the head opposite the injury, unroll the bandage around the head and below the eye against the cup. Then, wrap the bandage around the head and above the eye against the cup, completing a figure-8 pattern. Continue the same way, wrapping the bandage around the head and against the bottom of the cup *(above, left)*, then around the head and against the top of the cup. Finish wrapping the bandage with a final turn around the back of the head to the uninjured side, then tie the ends of it together *(above, right)*. Seek medical help immediately.

PREVENTING EYE AND EAR INJURIES

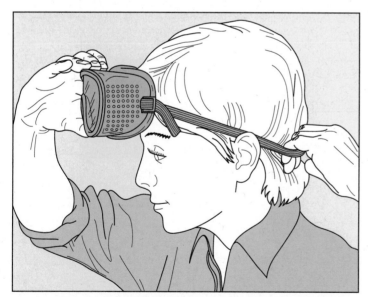

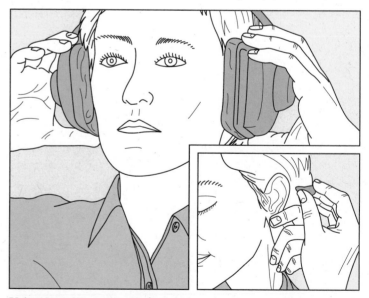

Using eye protection. To prevent an eye injury from flying dust or debris or a chemical splash when doing work around the house, wear safety goggles that are approved by the American National Standards Institute (ANSI) or the Canadian Standards Association (CSA). In general, use safety goggles with perforated vent holes *(above)* for protection from impact injury; with baffled vents for protection from chemical injury; with no vents for extremely dusty work or work using a chemical that emits irritating fumes. Never use safety goggles that are scratched, cracked or clouded. To use safety goggles, adjust the headstrap to seat them snugly against the face over the eyes.

Using hearing protection. To prevent hearing damage from high-intensity noise when using power tools, wear ear muffs; or, unless you have chronic ear problems, wear ear plugs. Use a device with a noise reduction rating (NRR) listed on its package; recommended is a device with a NRR of 25, which reduces noise by 25 decibels. To use ear muffs, adjust the headstrap to seat them snugly against the head over the ears *(above)*. To use foam ear plugs, ensure that your hands and the ear plugs are clean; roll each plug in turn between your fingers to compress it, then gently insert it into the ear canal *(inset)* and hold it in place until it expands to fit the shape of the canal.

BANDAGING THE EAR

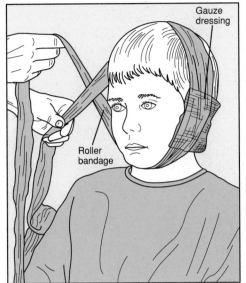
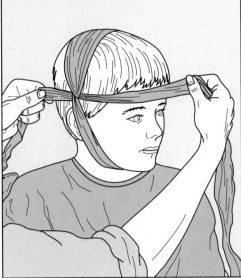
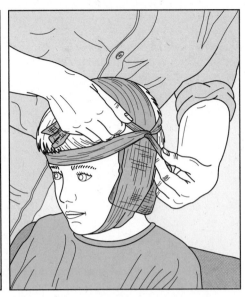

Bandaging a wounded outer ear. Have the victim sit still with his head upright. For a minor cut or scrape on the outer ear, wash the wound with soap and water, then cover it using an adhesive bandage. For a large wound on the outer ear, stop any bleeding by applying direct pressure using a sterile gauze dressing. If the dressing becomes blood-soaked, add another one over the first one; avoid lifting the dressing to inspect the wound. Continue applying direct pressure until the bleeding stops. If the bleeding persists or the wound is deep or gaping, seek medical help immediately. Otherwise, cover the wound with a clean gauze dressing. To hold the dressing in place on the wound, use a piece of gauze roller bandage about 3 feet long. Position the roller bandage with its midpoint against the dressing, then wrap it once around the head, drawing one end over the top and the other end under the chin to meet at the uninjured ear *(above, left)*. Twist one end of the roller bandage over the other end and pull the twist snug against the head *(above, center)*. Then, wrap the roller bandage back around the head, drawing one end around the front and one end around the back to tie them together above the injured ear *(above, right)*. Consult a physician if the wound becomes infected or any earache or hearing impairment follows the injury.

CLEARING AN OBJECT FROM THE EAR

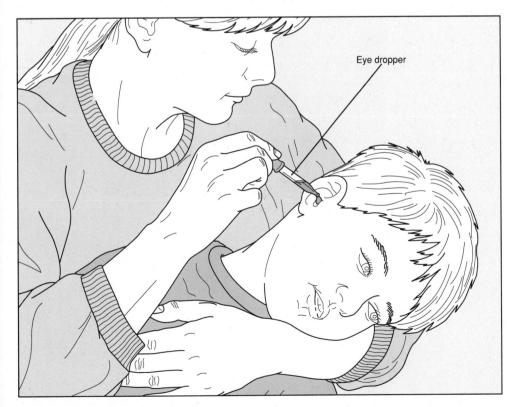

Dislodging an object from an ear.
Caution: Do not attempt to pull, pry or flush out an object lodged in the ear canal. Tilt the head on its side with the injured ear facing down, then shake the head slightly to dislodge the object. If you cannot dislodge an inanimate object from the ear, seek medical help immediately. If you cannot dislodge an insect from the ear, tilt the head on its side with the injured ear facing up and use an eye dropper to squeeze no more than 2 drops of mineral oil into the tip of the ear canal. Tilt the head on its side with the injured ear facing down and shake the head slightly to dislodge the insect. If you cannot dislodge the insect, seek medical help immediately. After dislodging an object from the ear, consult a physician if any earache or hearing impairment is experienced.

SKIN AND NAILS

Your skin is the covering that encloses all the other systems of the body. Not only does the skin protect the internal body parts from temperature fluctuations, impact injury and infection, but the sensory nerves in the skin provide the body with its vital sense of touch. The diagram on page 101 illustrates the anatomy of a typical section of skin and its internal components. The skin itself is comprised of three layers: an outer cell layer (epidermis); a middle layer containing blood vessels (dermis); and an inner subcutaneous layer attached to the muscles and bones. Nerve endings called receptors are scattered throughout the dermis and provide the skin with its sensitivity to heat, cold, pressure and pain. Sebaceous glands in hair-bearing areas of the skin secrete oils that keep the skin supple; sweat glands secrete liquids that cool the skin in response to heat. The nails are a specialized, translucent form of the epidermis that covers the dermis of the fingertips and toes.

Due to their constant exposure to the external environment, the skin and nails of the body are vulnerable to many types of injuries and infections. While most disorders of the skin and nails are not serious, even a minor problem with them can cause considerable distress—due to the major role that they often play in a person's appearance and sense of well-being. Any itching, swelling or pain of the skin or nails can be extremely bothersome, but is rarely a symptom of a serious disorder. Any new growth on the skin, however, should be taken seriously and reported to a physician as soon as possible. The health tips at right cover basic guidelines for keeping the skin, nails and hair healthy.

The Troubleshooting Guide on page 102 puts procedures for common skin, nail and hair disorders at your fingertips and refers you to pages 103 to 109 for more detailed information. Familiarize yourself with the procedures for treating injuries to the skin such as a cut, scrape or puncture *(page 103)*, an insect bite or sting or a splinter *(page 104)*, a snakebite *(page 105)*, a burn *(page 106)*, a poison plant irritation *(page 107)* and frostbite *(page 107)*. Know how to relieve pressure from an ingrown toenail *(page 108)* and how to treat a corn or callus *(page 109)*. For techniques on handling a life-threatening emergency such as severe bleeding, a severe or extensive burn, or hypothermia, refer to the Emergency Guide *(page 8)*. For basic techniques on caring for a family member who is ill or recuperating from an illness, consult the Equipment & Techniques chapter *(page 110)*.

If you must cope with a disorder of the skin, nails or hair, do not hesitate to call for help; medical professionals can answer questions about symptoms and treatments. Post the telephone numbers for your physician, local hospital emergency room, ambulance and pharmacy near the telephone; in most regions, dial 911 in the event of a life-threatening emergency. Keep on hand the telephone number of a dermatologist recommended by your physician.

HEALTH TIPS

1. To help keep your skin, nails and hair healthy, eat a well-balanced diet; practice proper hygiene and good grooming.

2. Avoid using scented soaps that dry the skin; many contain ingredients that deplete skin of its natural oils. Use soaps with oatmeal or lipid-free lotions, or super-fatted soaps.

3. To prevent dry skin, avoid using extremely hot water when bathing. Dry the skin thoroughly after bathing; if necessary, apply a moisturizer, especially to the skin of the feet.

4. To prevent sun damage to the skin, always apply a sunscreen before exposure to the sun. Avoid exposure to the sun at mid-day when its ultraviolet radiation is strongest.

5. Avoid the use of tanning salons and tanning lights unless your physician recommends it; tanning lights can be as damaging to the skin as strong sunlight if used improperly.

6. Protect the skin in cold weather by dressing properly for it in layers of loose clothing. Take special care with the areas of the body where heat loss is greatest: the head, chest, armpits and groin. The skin of the face, hands and feet is especially susceptible to frostbite.

7. To prevent injury to the skin of your hands, wear work gloves when handling rough or sharp objects; wear heavy-duty rubber gloves when handling caustic chemicals. Protect the skin of your arms and legs by wearing a long-sleeved shirt and long pants.

8. To prevent a fungal infection of the feet such as athlete's foot, regularly wash and dry the feet well, especially between the toes. Wear socks of absorbent cotton or wool; avoid materials of synthetic fibers.

9. Protect the nails by keeping them trimmed and clean, using cosmetic preparations sparingly, and keeping exposure to water at a minimum. In particular, keep the nails of a child trimmed short to discourage nail-biting and the spread of infection from dirt under the nails.

10. To prevent ingrown toenails, cut the nails straight across; do not shape the edges of them. Wear shoes that fit properly and do not cramp the toes.

11. Consult a physician about any potentially-serious symptom of a skin problem such as an unusual growth and any extensive or recurring rash, swelling or blistering.

12. To prevent the spread of contagious skin and hair infections, do not share facecloths, towels, combs or hairbrushes.

13. Carefully follow the physician's directions to use any prescription medication for a skin, nail or hair; use only the amount specified at only the prescribed times and report any side effect to the physician.

14. To use a nonprescription skin medication to treat a minor skin problem such as dryness or itchiness, carefully follow the manufacturer's directions.

SKIN

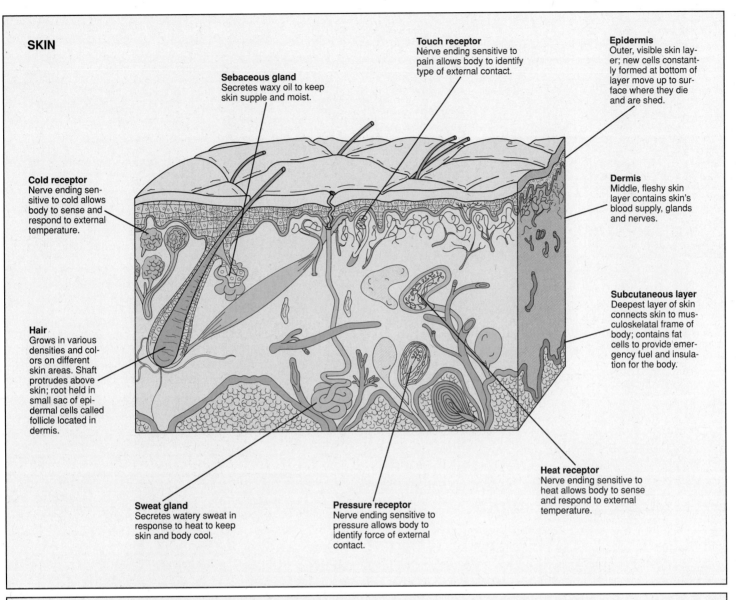

Sebaceous gland
Secretes waxy oil to keep skin supple and moist.

Touch receptor
Nerve ending sensitive to pain allows body to identify type of external contact.

Epidermis
Outer, visible skin layer; new cells constantly formed at bottom of layer move up to surface where they die and are shed.

Cold receptor
Nerve ending sensitive to cold allows body to sense and respond to external temperature.

Dermis
Middle, fleshy skin layer contains skin's blood supply, glands and nerves.

Subcutaneous layer
Deepest layer of skin connects skin to musculoskelatal frame of body; contains fat cells to provide emergency fuel and insulation for the body.

Hair
Grows in various densities and colors on different skin areas. Shaft protrudes above skin; root held in small sac of epidermal cells called follicle located in dermis.

Sweat gland
Secretes watery sweat in response to heat to keep skin and body cool.

Pressure receptor
Nerve ending sensitive to pressure allows body to identify force of external contact.

Heat receptor
Nerve ending sensitive to heat allows body to sense and respond to external temperature.

NAIL

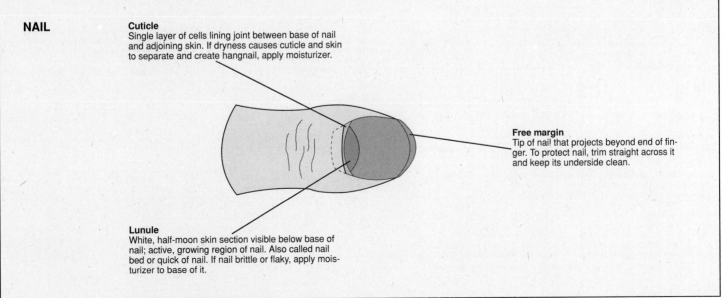

Cuticle
Single layer of cells lining joint between base of nail and adjoining skin. If dryness causes cuticle and skin to separate and create hangnail, apply moisturizer.

Free margin
Tip of nail that projects beyond end of finger. To protect nail, trim straight across it and keep its underside clean.

Lunule
White, half-moon skin section visible below base of nail; active, growing region of nail. Also called nail bed or quick of nail. If nail brittle or flaky, apply moisturizer to base of it.

TROUBLESHOOTING GUIDE

PROBLEM	PROCEDURE
Cut or scrape	Treat cut or scrape (p. 103)
	Consult a physician for tetanus treatment if wound caused by rusty or dirty object
Splinter	Remove splinter (p. 104)
Puncture of skin	Treat puncture (p. 103)
	Consult a physician for tetanus treatment if wound caused by rusty or dirty object
Object embedded in skin	Stabilize embedded object (p. 105) and seek emergency help ✚
Insect bite or sting	Treat insect bite or sting (p. 104)
	Seek emergency help ✚ if victim suffers severe allergic reaction; if necessary, use emergency first aid (p. 8)
Animal bite	Seek emergency help ✚ if bleeding severe, or wound deep or gaping
	Treat cut, scrape or puncture (p. 103)
	Consult a physician for tetanus or rabies treatment
Snakebite	Treat snakebite (p. 105)
	Seek emergency help ✚ if victim suffers difficulty breathing, weakness, swelling or vomiting; if necessary, use emergency first aid (p. 8)
Burn	Seek emergency help ✚ if burn severe; if necessary, use emergency first aid (p. 8)
	Treat burn (p. 106)
Sunburn	Seek emergency help ✚ if burn severe; if necessary, use emergency first aid (p. 8)
	Treat burn and prevent sunburn (p. 106)
Poison plant irritation	Treat poison plant irritation (p. 107)
Frostbite	Seek emergency help ✚ if frostbite severe; if necessary, use emergency first aid (p. 8)
	Treat frostbite (p. 107)
Ingrown toenail	Treat ingrown toenail (p. 108)
Corn or callus	Treat corn or callus (p. 109)
Athlete's foot suspected: soggy, flaking, itchy skin between toes or on soles of feet	Keep skin clean and dry; use nonprescription skin medication (p. 108) and avoid scratching
	Consult a physician if problem severe or persists
Psoriasis suspected: red, scaly eruption	Consult a physician
Impetigo suspected: yellow, crusty eruption	Consult a physician
Wart	Keep skin clean and dry; use nonprescription wart medication and avoid picking
	Consult a physician if problem severe or persists
Blackhead or pimple	Keep skin clean and dry; use nonprescription skin medication (p. 108) and avoid picking
	Consult a physician if problem severe or persists
Blister	Cover blister with sterile gauze dressing; avoid breaking
	Consult a physician if blister becomes inflamed, swollen or pus-filled
Bruise	Consult a physician if bruise not due to impact injury
	Administer cold treatment (p. 120) for 15 to 20 minutes every few hours for 48 hours
	Consult a physician if pain or swelling lasts more than 3 days, or discoloration or tenderness lasts more than 3 weeks
Open sore	Keep skin clean and dry; avoid picking
	Consult a physician if sore accompanied by pain or bleeding, or does not heal in 5 days
Lump, bump, cyst or mole	Consult a physician if growth on breast or genitals, develops rapidly, or painful or bleeds
Rash	Consult a physician
Skin dry, rough or itchy	Use nonprescription skin medication (p. 108); consult a physician if problem severe or persists
Hair dry or thinning; scalp flaky or itchy	Maintain healthy hair (p. 109); consult a physician if problem severe or persists

✚ Medical emergency

TREATING A CUT OR SCRAPE

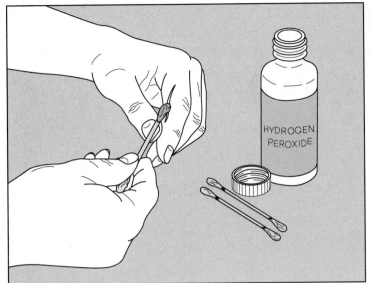

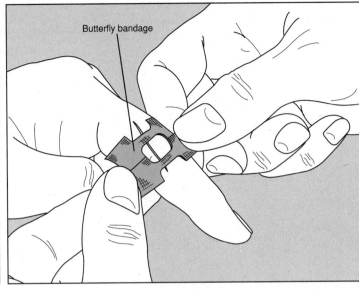

Butterfly bandage

Cleaning and bandaging a wound. For a wound caused by a rusty or dirty object, consult a physician for treatment for possible tetanus. To stop any bleeding, elevate the wound and apply direct pressure to it using a sterile gauze dressing. If the dressing becomes blood-soaked, add another one over the first one; avoid lifting the dressing to inspect the wound. If the bleeding persists or the wound is deep or gaping, seek emergency help immediately. Otherwise, clean the wound by washing it gently using soap and water; or, apply hydrogen peroxide to it using a clean cotton swab *(above, left)*. Leave a minor scrape uncovered to pro-

mote healing; avoid getting it dirty until it heals. For a small cut, apply an adhesive bandage; if the wound has well-defined edges, use a butterfly bandage that holds its edges together and leaves the rest of it exposed to air *(above, right)*. Cover a large wound by applying a gauze dressing; wrap the dressing with a gauze roller bandage and secure the roller bandage with adhesive tape. Remove any bandage after 24 to 48 hours. Consult a physician if the wound shows any sign of infection—such as inflammation, swelling, pain or pus.

TREATING A PUNCTURE

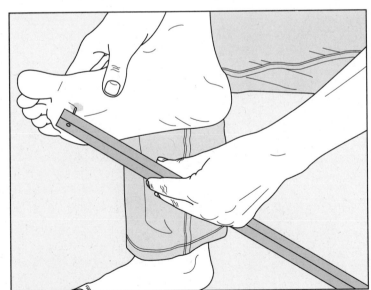

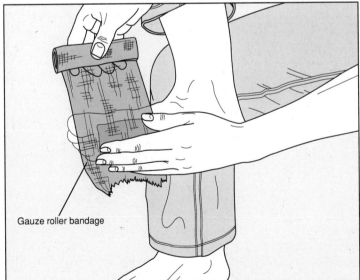

Gauze roller bandage

Cleaning and bandaging a wound. For a puncture caused by a rusty or dirty object, consult a physician for treatment for possible tetanus. If the object is deeply embedded in the skin, do not remove it; stabilize it *(page 105)* and seek emergency help. Otherwise, gently remove the object from the skin *(above, left)*, then let the wound bleed freely for several minutes to help clean it. To stop the bleeding, elevate the wound and apply direct pressure to it using a sterile gauze dressing. If the dressing becomes blood-soaked, add another one over the first one; avoid lifting the dressing to inspect the wound. If the bleeding

persists or the wound is deep or gaping, seek emergency help immediately. Otherwise, clean the wound by washing it gently using soap and water; or, apply hydrogen peroxide to it using a clean cotton swab. To prevent infection, apply a gauze dressing to the wound, then wrap the dressing with a gauze roller bandage *(above, right)* and secure the roller bandage with adhesive tape. Remove any bandage after 24 to 48 hours. Consult a physician if the wound shows any sign of infection—such as inflammation, swelling, pain or pus.

TREATING AN INSECT BITE OR STING

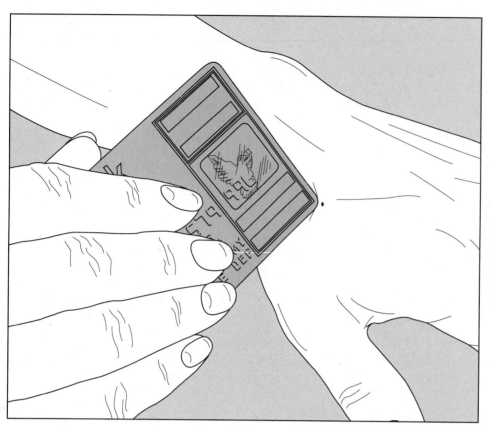

Relieving pain and itching. Remove any bee stinger and sac immediately. **Caution:** Do not use tweezers; they can squeeze additional venom from the sac into the victim. Use a credit card to scrape the stinger and sac off the skin *(left)*. Or, if the stinger and sac are embedded in the skin, work them out using the tip of a needle sterilized over a flame or in rubbing alcohol. Wash the skin with soap and water. To reduce any pain or swelling of the skin, apply an ice pack or a plastic bag of ice cubes wrapped in a towel. Monitor the victim for signs of an allergic reaction *(page 25)*. To relieve any itching of the skin, use a cotton ball to dab it with hydrocortisone cream or calamine lotion, or apply a paste of sodium bicarbonate (baking soda) and water; do not scratch the skin. Consult a physician if the itching does not subside in 2 to 3 days. If necessary, consult a physician about an allergy test and allergy shots; if recommended, buy an emergency kit for use in treating an allergic reaction in the future.

REMOVING A SPLINTER

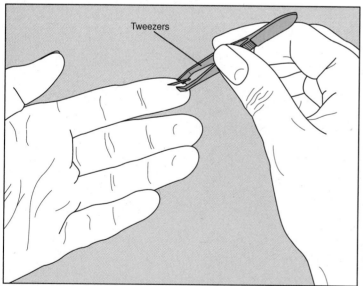

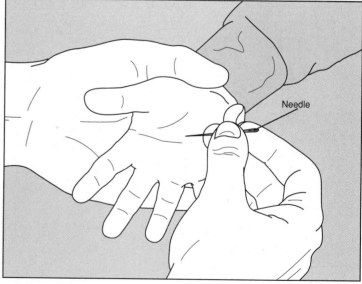

Pulling out a splinter. Wash the skin around the splinter with soap and water. A metal splinter may require a treatment for tetanus; consult a physician. Otherwise, sterilize the ends of tweezers in rubbing alcohol or over a flame and wipe them using a piece of sterile gauze; for an embedded splinter, also sterilize the tip of a needle the same way. To remove a protruding splinter, grasp the end of it with the tweezers and gently pull it out *(above, left)*. To remove an embedded splinter, first ease it out from under the skin using the tip of the needle *(above, right)*, then pull it out with the tweezers. Wash the wound with soap and water. Consult a physician if you cannot remove the splinter or the wound shows any sign of infection—such as inflammation, swelling, pain or pus.

TREATING A SNAKEBITE

Monitoring a snakebite victim. Most snakes in the U.S. are not poisonous; the victim of a snakebite may experience no more than its initial pinch. A snakebite from a rattlesnake or a copperhead, water-moccasin or coral snake, however, can constitute a serious medical emergency; in 70 percent of these snakebites, venom is injected—in an amount that depends on the size of the snake. Although a lethal amount of venom is seldom injected, treat any potentially-poisonous snakebite as serious; seek emergency help immediately. Blood is usually present around a snakebite and it may not clot if venom has been injected. To limit the poisoning effects of venom, assist the snakebite victim *(step right)*. If venom has not been injected with the snakebite, no symptoms should develop; otherwise, be alert to signs of an emergency:

- Extreme pain and swelling around the snakebite

- Shallow or uneven breathing *(page 12)*

- Slow, rapid or irregular pulse *(page 13)*

- Physical weakness or numbness

- Nausea or vomiting

- Visual disturbances

- Shock *(page 23)*

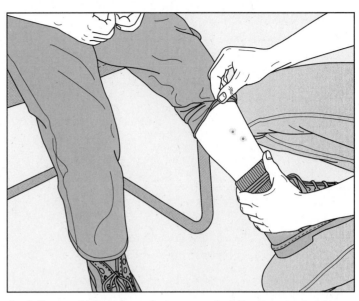

Assisting a victim of a poisonous snakebite. Do not administer any nonprescription pain-reliever to the victim. Call for emergency help, then have the victim rest comfortably, keeping the injury below the level of his heart, if possible. Remove any footwear, jewelry or clothing from the injured area *(above)*. For a snakebite on a limb, limit the poisoning effects of any venom by restricting the flow of blood to and from the snakebite. Tie a cloth strip or belt around the limb 4 inches from each side of the snakebite; tie it tight enough for a finger to fit under it and loosen it if any swelling occurs. Keep the victim calm and quiet until emergency help arrives.

STABILIZING AN OBJECT EMBEDDED IN THE SKIN

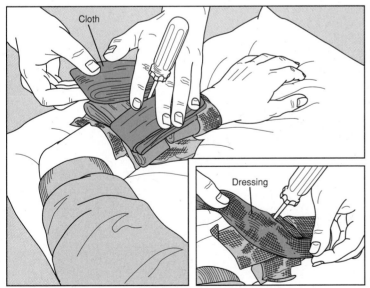

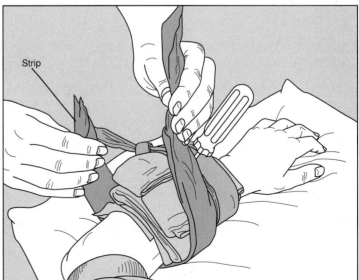

Immobilizing an embedded object. Caution: Do not attempt to pull out the embedded object; if it protrudes from the skin, immobilize it to prevent further injury and control any bleeding. Have the victim sit or lie still and elevate the injury. Place sterile gauze dressings on the injury around the embedded object *(inset)*; do not apply pressure on the embedded object. Then, build a support around the embedded object by packing clean, folded cloths or feminine napkins around the base of it *(above, left)*. To secure the support, use cloths folded into strips or strips of gauze roller bandage. Wrap each strip around the injury on opposite sides of the embedded object *(above, right)* and tie its ends together into a knot. Seek emergency help immediately.

TREATING A BURN

Treating a burn. A burn is an injury to the skin tissue that may result from exposure to heat, a chemical, the sun, a hot liquid or steam, electrical current or lightning. The severity of a burn depends on its surface area and depth: a first-degree burn may cause reddening of the skin; a second-degree burn may cause the skin to turn red and blister; a third-degree burn may result in dry, pale-white skin or brown, charred skin.

By acting quickly *(step right)*, the pain and scarring of a burn can be lessened. Treat a burn following the precautions listed below:

• Seek emergency help immediately for any burn larger in size than the victim's hand or to the face or genitals.

• Remove clothing, jewelry and footwear from a burn before any swelling begins; leave clothing adhered to it.

• Do not apply any antiseptic spray or ointment to a burn; never apply a moisturizing lotion, butter, margarine or oil.

• Do not apply a chemical neutralizer such as vinegar, baking soda or alcohol to a chemical burn.

• To help prevent infection, do not touch a burn; also avoid breathing, coughing or sneezing on it. Never break the blisters of a burn.

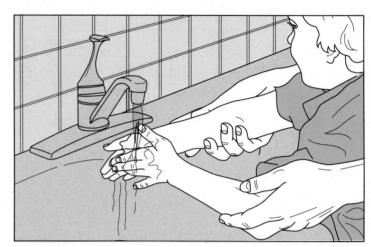

Treating a burn victim. Gently remove any clothing, jewelry and footwear from the burn; do not attempt to remove clothing adhered to it. For a burn due to a chemical powder, use a clean, dry cloth to lightly brush any powder off the skin. If the burn is severe, cover it lightly with a sterile gauze dressing and seek emergency help immediately. Otherwise, immerse the burn in cold water, flushing it with a gentle flow of cool water from a faucet *(above)*, shower head or garden hose. Flush the burn for at least 15 minutes or until any pain subsides, then gently pat it dry; repeat the procedure as often as necessary to relieve discomfort. Until the burn heals, rest and keep it elevated as much as possible; drink plenty of fluids.

PREVENTING SUNBURN

Protecting the skin from the sun. Contrary to popular belief, there is no such thing as a healthy tan. Any person, regardless of skin type, should avoid unnecessary exposure to the sun. Excess exposure to sunlight in summer or winter can cause sunburn. While minor sunburn causes redness and slight pain of the skin, sometimes accompanied by its peeling, severe sunburn can cause blistering and other damage to the skin, as well as serious illness.

• If a sunburn causes fluid-filled blistering of the skin, fever, visual disturbances or dizziness, seek medical help immediately.

• If you have a sunburn, stay out of the sun until the skin heals. To relieve discomfort, soak in a bathtub of cool water; add 1/2 cup of sodium bicarbonate (baking soda) to the water.

• A fair-skinned person is most prone to sunburn and should expose the skin to the sun only gradually.

• To tan without a sunburn, start with a few minutes of exposure to the sun each day, allowing the skin to build up its own sun protection; gradually increase time spent in the sun.

• For sensitive skin, use a sunscreen designed to block out ultraviolet radiation. Choose a physical sunscreen such as zinc oxide to prevent tanning and sunburn; choose a chemical sunscreen to allow tanning and prevent sunburn.

Repeated sunburn can eventually cause permanent damage to skin tissue, making it leathery and dry. Also, many skin cancers can be traced to repeated, prolonged exposure to the ultraviolet rays of the sun. Melanoma, an often fatal form of skin cancer, can result from repeated short periods of exposure to intense sunlight over years. Refer to the guidelines below to help you guard your skin against overexposure to the sun:

• When choosing a chemical sunscreen, look for a product with a sun protection factor (SPF) rating on the label; recommended by many dermatologists is an SPF rating of at least 15.

• Check the product label of a chemical sunscreen to determine the active ingredient; recommended is a product with an active ingredient of aminobenzoic acid (PABA), cinoxate, oxybenzone or padimate O.

• For maximum skin protection, prepare it 40 to 60 minutes before going into the sun. Clean and dry the skin, then apply a sunscreen to it following the manufacturer's instructions. To protect the lips, apply a lip balm that has an SPF rating.

• Reapply a sunscreen periodically during any prolonged exposure to sunlight, especially after swimming or any physical activity that causes perspiration; make sure that the skin is thoroughly dry before reapplying the sunscreen.

TREATING A POISONOUS PLANT IRRITATION

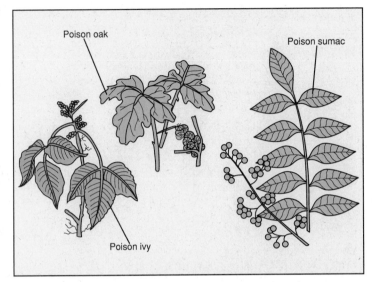

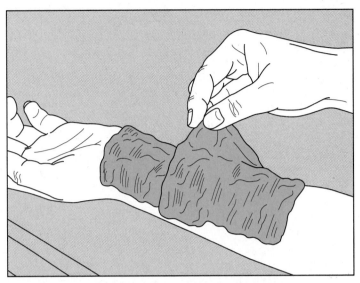

Identifying poisonous plants. A poisonous plant can grow as a bush, climbing vine, shrub or small tree. Poison ivy and poison oak can be identified by their leaves; only one leaf composed of three leaflets grows from each stem node, the center leaflet having the longest stem. Poison ivy leaflets are oval, tapered to a point *(above, left)* and red in spring. Poison oak leaflets are rounder, lobed like oak leaves *(above, center)*, hairy on the top and velvety on the bottom. Poison ivy and poison oak may have greenish flowers in late spring and berries later; poison ivy berries remain all winter. Posion sumac *(above, right)* grows as a shrub or small tree from 5 to 25 feet tall.

Treating skin irritation from a poisonous plant. Contact with a poisonous plant can irritate the skin, causing an itchy rash. Remove any clothing from the irritated skin and wash with soap and water; also wash any clothing in contact with the poisonous plant. To reduce itching, use a cotton ball to dab the irritated skin with hydrocortisone cream or calamine lotion; or, cover the irritated skin using gauze dressings soaked with cool water *(above)*. The itchiness should subside in 2 to 3 days. Do not scratch the skin; to prevent a child from scratching himself, trim his fingernails. Consult a physician if any swelling, blistering or itchiness lasts more than 1 week.

TREATING FROSTBITE

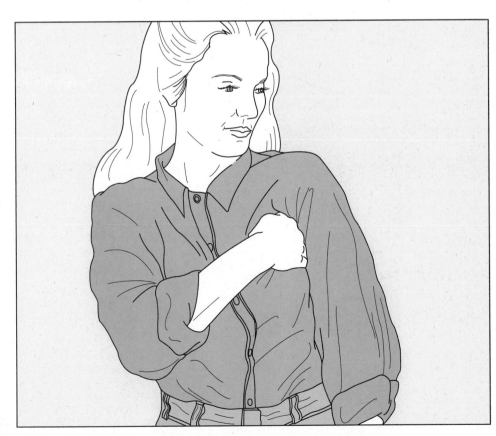

Treating a frostbite victim. Unprotected skin exposed to extreme cold and high wind may become numb and white, symptoms of frostbite; the nose, ears, face, hands and feet are especially susceptible. **Caution:** Do not rub or walk on frostbitten skin; crystallized moisture in it can cause severe injury. Move the victim indoors and keep him warm. Gently remove any clothing, jewelry or footwear from the skin to examine it. Frostbite is classified by degrees of severity: first-degree frostbite may cause reddish skin and a prickly, burning sensation; second-degree frostbite may cause blistered or mottled gray skin and a prickly, burning sensation that leads to numbness; third-degree frostbite may cause shiny-white, leathery skin and numbness. Seek emergency help immediately if the frostbite is severe. Otherwise, allow the frostbitten skin to warm gradually, warming it with heat from your hands or armpits *(left)* or by immersing it in a bucket or basin of tepid water. **Caution:** Do not immerse frostbitten skin in hot water or apply direct heat. After warming the skin, apply a gauze dressing and secure it with adhesive tape. Consult a physician if any discoloration, prickly or burning sensation, or loss of sensation lasts more than 1 day.

USING NONPRESCRIPTION SKIN MEDICATIONS

PRODUCT	APPLICATION
Antibiotic	Cream or gel for preventing infection of cut or scrape; apply directly to wound
Antiseptic	Cream or gel for cleaning cut or scrape; apply directly to wound
Bath oil	Oil for moisturizing dry, chapped skin; mix with bath water or apply directly to skin
Benzoyl peroxide; retinoic acid	Lotion, cream or gel for preventing infection or drying of blemish; apply directly to skin
Calamine	Lotion for relieving itching; apply directly to skin
Cocoa butter	Lotion, cream, oil or gel for moisturizing dry, chapped skin; apply directly to skin
Cornstarch	Powder for drying chapped skin or controlling fungal infection; apply directly to skin
Glycerin	Lotion for moisturizing dry, chapped skin; apply directly to skin
Hydrocortisone; hydrocortisone acetate	Cream for relieving itching; apply directly to skin
Petrolatum	Lotion for moisturizing dry, chapped skin; apply directly to wet skin after soaking in water
Sodium bicarbonate (baking soda)	Powder for relieving itching; mix with water into paste and apply directly to skin or into solution and soak skin
Talcum powder	Powder for drying chapped skin or controlling fungal infection; apply directly to skin
Urea; lactic acid	Lotion for moisturizing dry, chapped skin; apply directly to skin
Zinc oxide	Cream for relieving itching; apply directly to skin

Choosing a skin-care product. For a severe or extensive skin irritation, consult a physician. To treat everyday dryness or itchiness of the skin and minor skin irritations due to heat, friction or moisture, many nonprescription skin medications are available at any pharmacy. Consult the chart at left to identify the type of product or active ingredient of a product that is best suited to your skin problem. Always carefully read the label of any product you buy to ensure that it can be used for your particular skin problem; pay special attention to any warnings or information on possible side effects. If you are in doubt about a product, ask the pharmacist for advice. Follow the manufacturer's instructions for any product, using only the amount specified at the proper times. If a product aggravates a skin problem, discontinue your use of it and consult a physician.

TREATING AN INGROWN TOENAIL

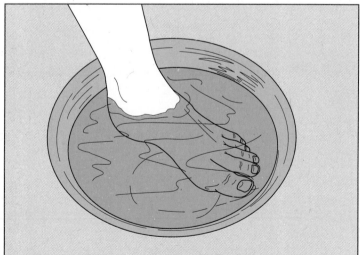

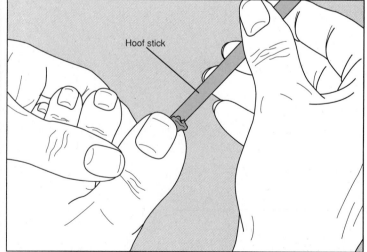

Hoof stick

Relieving pressure on an ingrown toenail. Consult a physician about an ingrown toenail if you are diabetic or the toe is swollen, painful or bleeding. Otherwise, treat the ingrown toenail yourself by soaking and dressing it twice a day to relieve the pressure on it. Fill a basin or bucket with warm water and soak the toe *(above, left)* for 15 to 20 minutes, softening the skin around the toenail. Thoroughly dry the foot with a clean towel. Cut a small piece of gauze dressing and wrap it around

the pointed end of a hoof stick, then coat it with a small amount of a nonprescription antiseptic or antibiotic ointment. Use the hoofstick to gently lift the ingrown toenail and insert the dressing under it *(above, right)*. Leave the dressing in place until you are ready to soak the toe and dress the toenail again. Consult a physician if home treatment does not clear up the problem after 1 week. Prevent an ingrown toenail with proper care of the feet *(page 47)*.

TREATING A CORN OR CALLUS

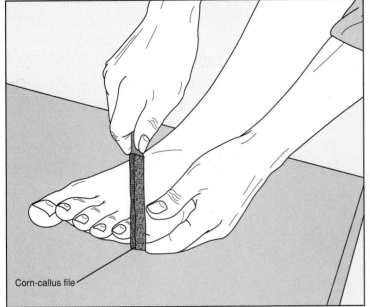

Corn-callus file

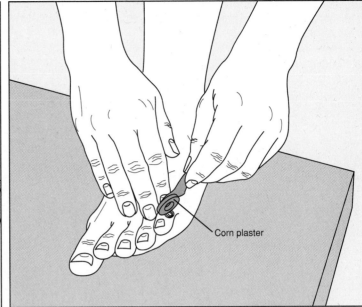

Corn plaster

Relieving pressure on a corn or a callus. Consult a physician about a corn if you are diabetic or it is painful, bleeding or infected. Otherwise, treat a corn or callus yourself by soaking and paring it daily. Fill a basin or bucket with warm water and soak the toe for 15 to 20 minutes to soften the skin, then thoroughly dry it with a clean towel. To pare a corn or callus, use a pumice stone or a corn-callus file. Working only in one direction, gently draw the stone or file repeatedly across the surface of the corn or callus *(above, left)*, smoothing it level with the surrounding skin. To help relieve pressure on a corn when wearing shoes, apply a commercial corn plaster on it *(above, right)*. Consult a physician if home treatment does not clear up the problem after 1 week. Prevent a corn or callus with proper care of the feet *(page 47)*.

MAINTAINING HEALTHY HAIR

Preventing hair damage. Constant exposure to water, sunlight, detergents and manipulation by brushing and hairdressing exacts a toll on even the healthiest head of hair. With time and age, some discoloration, thinning and loss of hair is inevitable. As well, the metabolic changes that accompany conditions such as a prolonged or serious illness, childbirth, contraceptive usage or dieting can affect the health and condition of the hair. In some cases, however, premature hair loss may be due to a disorder that can be treated with medication. Consult a physician if any problem of the hair or scalp is persistent and worsens over time or causes any degree of discomfort or embarrassment. Follow the guidelines below to maintain healthy hair and prevent damage that can lead to hair loss:

• To encourage normal hair growth, eat a well-balanced diet that supplies all the vitamins, minerals and proteins necessary for healthy hair production.

• Avoid over-brushing the hair; following the conventional wisdom to give the hair "100 brushstrokes per night" can roughen and otherwise damage the hair.

• To brush tangled hair, use a vulcanized sawtooth comb—not a brush—to gently smooth out the tangles.

• Many commercial shampoos are advertised as effective for dry, normal or oily hair; in general, choose a shampoo that is labeled as mild and leaves your hair looking and feeling clean.

• If you suffer from dandruff, use a nonprescription medicated shampoo that contains an active ingredient such as zinc pyrithione, salicylic acid or sulfur, or a nonmedicated shampoo containing a surfactant or detergent. Consult a physician if a dandruff problem is persistent or embarrassing.

• In general, wash the hair thoroughly every 2 to 3 days. Wet your hair with warm, clean water and rub a few drops of shampoo into it, then rinse it well and repeat. To apply a conditioner to the hair, let it sit for the length of time specified by the manufacturer. Gently pat the hair dry with a clean towel.

• When using a hair dryer, avoid selecting a heat setting higher than medium and do not handle the hair excessively while it is hot. Keep the dryer nozzle at least 6 inches from the hair and move it constantly while drying the hair. Ensure that a hair dryer is Underwriters Laboratories (UL) approved.

• To prevent damage to the hair, minimize the use of hairdressing techniques such as tight braiding, curling with heated tongs or rollers, and bleaching, dyeing or perming.

• If you swim regularly in a chlorinated swimming pool, minimize hair exposure to chlorine by wearing a bathing cap. Many hair care salons and swimming pools sell anti-chlorine hair treatment products; follow the manufacturer's instructions to use one.

EQUIPMENT & TECHNIQUES

This section introduces basic equipment and techniques for family medical care at home. You can handle most family medical care at home with the kit of equipment and supplies shown below and on page 111. Basic items such as dressings and bandages, toothpaste and dental floss, and a reusable hot or cold compress can be purchased at a local pharmacy; for a specialized item such as a blood-pressure monitoring device or a tooth preserving kit, you may need to go to a medical supply center or consult your physician or dentist. For guidance on the safe use of nonprescription pain-relievers and other medication, refer to the information presented on pages 121 to 122.

With routine physical checkups, many family medical problems can be prevented; and problems that may arise can be easier to treat if they are detected in their early stages. Establish an ongoing relationship with a physician with whom you feel comfortable *(page 125)* and follow his recommendations on scheduled medical examinations and tests *(page 124)*. Avert the financial hardship entailed in the event of a medical problem requiring expensive diagnosis or treatment by setting up a suitable plan of medical insurance coverage *(page 125)*. Refer to the Emergency Guide *(page 8)* for information on identifying and handling a family medical emergency.

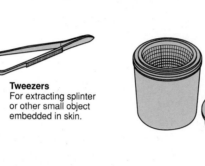

Safety pins
For securing bandage; available in variety of shapes and sizes.

Tweezers
For extracting splinter or other small object embedded in skin.

Tooth preserving kit
For storing tooth knocked out of gum; preserves tooth for reimplanting by dentist for up to 12 hours.

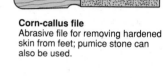

Corn-callus file
Abrasive file for removing hardened skin from feet; pumice stone can also be used.

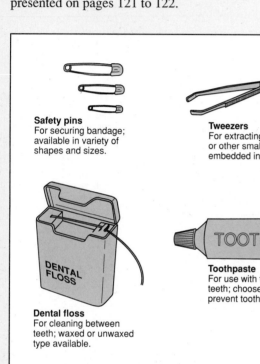

Dental floss
For cleaning between teeth; waxed or unwaxed type available.

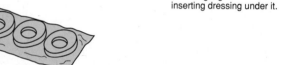

Toothpaste
For use with toothbrush to clean teeth; choose fluoride type to help prevent tooth decay.

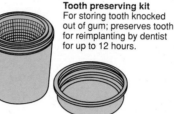

Corn plasters
Non-medicated adhesive pad for relieving pressure on corn exerted by shoe.

Hoof stick
For lifting ingrown toenail and inserting dressing under it.

Emery board
Tapered end for cleaning free margin of nails; blunted end for easing cuticles off lunules of nails.

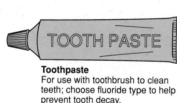

Toothbrush
For use with toothpaste to clean teeth; unless otherwise recommended by dentist, choose type with soft bristles.

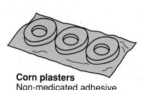

Eye dropper
Calibrated tube for administering measured doses of liquid medication.

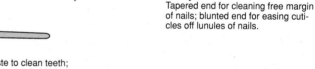

Medication spoon
Calibrated tube for administering exact dosage of liquid medication.

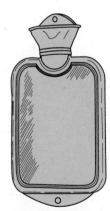

Hot-water bottle
For relieving discomfort of strain or sprain of muscle or joint or other minor injury; heating pad can also be used.

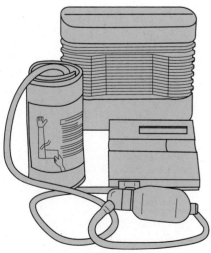

Blood-pressure monitoring device
For home-monitoring of blood pressure: electronic type shown provides reading on liquid crystal display; older type provides reading on calibrated pressure gauge.

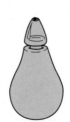

Nasal aspirator
For removing mucus from nose of infant.

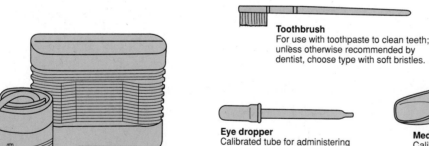

Reusable hot or cold compress
For relieving discomfort of headache, strain or sprain of muscle or joint, or other minor injury.

Caring at home for a family member who is ill or recuperating from an illness need not be a strenuous ordeal; often, only a few simple techniques are needed. Be familiar with the ways of monitoring temperature *(page 114)* and taking a pulse *(page 115)*. Set up a recovery room to make a patient as comfortable as possible *(page 112)*. Know how to move a patient, assisting him in turning over or sitting up in bed, or in getting out of bed to sit on a chair *(page 116)*. Bathe a patient who is confined to bed *(page 118)*. To help relieve a patient of discomfort, administer cold *(page 120)* and heat *(page 119)* treatments. Know how to change a bandage *(page 123)*.

Never hesitate to obtain medical help when you need it. Consult your physician if you ever have questions about the care of a family member who is ill or recuperating from an illness, or if the signs and symptoms of a potential medical problem change or persist. Ask your physician or pharmacist for instructions on administering any prescribed medication and for possible side effects to monitor; report any side effects that occur to your physician. Keep the telephone numbers for your physician, local hospital emergency room, ambulance and pharmacy posted near the telephone; in most regions, dial 911 in the event of a life-threatening emergency.

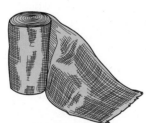

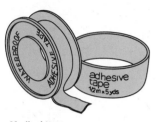

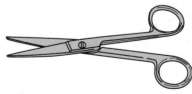

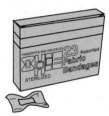

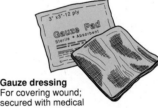

Roller bandage
For applying compression to strained or sprained muscle or joint.

Adhesive bandages
Gauze dressing with adhesive strip for protecting minor cut or scratch; available in variety of shapes and sizes.

Medical tape
For securing dressing; hypo-allergenic type available for sensitive skin.

Gauze roller bandage
For securing gauze dressing; roll about 5 yards long available in 2-inch or 3-inch width.

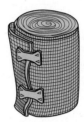

Triangular bandage
Multipurpose bandage can be folded for making sling, swathe, ring pad or head bandage, for example; measures about 55 inches along base and 36 to 40 inches on each other side.

Gauze dressing
For covering wound; secured with medical tape or gauze roller bandage. Available in 2-by-2 inch, 3-by-3 inch, or 4-by-4 inch sizes.

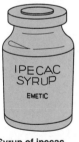

Cotton balls
For applying soothing medication such as hydrocortisone cream or calamine lotion; also for cleaning of genitals before collecting urine sample.

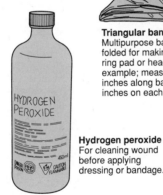

Hydrogen peroxide
For cleaning wound before applying dressing or bandage.

Nail clippers
For trimming nails of fingers and toes; cut toenails straight across to prevent them from becoming ingrown.

Syrup of ipecac
For inducing vomiting in victim of ingested poisoning. **Caution:** Administer only if advised by poison control center or physician.

Isopropyl (rubbing) alcohol
For sterilizing needle, tweezers and other first-aid equipment.

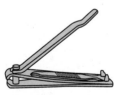

Scissors
For cutting medical tape, gauze roller bandage and other items.

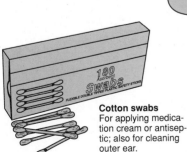

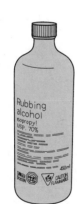

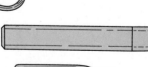

Petroleum jelly
For moisturizing dry, chapped skin; also for lubricating bulb of thermometer before taking rectal temperature.

Cotton swabs
For applying medication cream or antiseptic; also for cleaning outer ear.

Thermometer
For determining body temperature: electronic type shown provides reading on liquid crystal display; older type provides reading on calibrated vial of mercury.

SETTING UP A RECOVERY ROOM

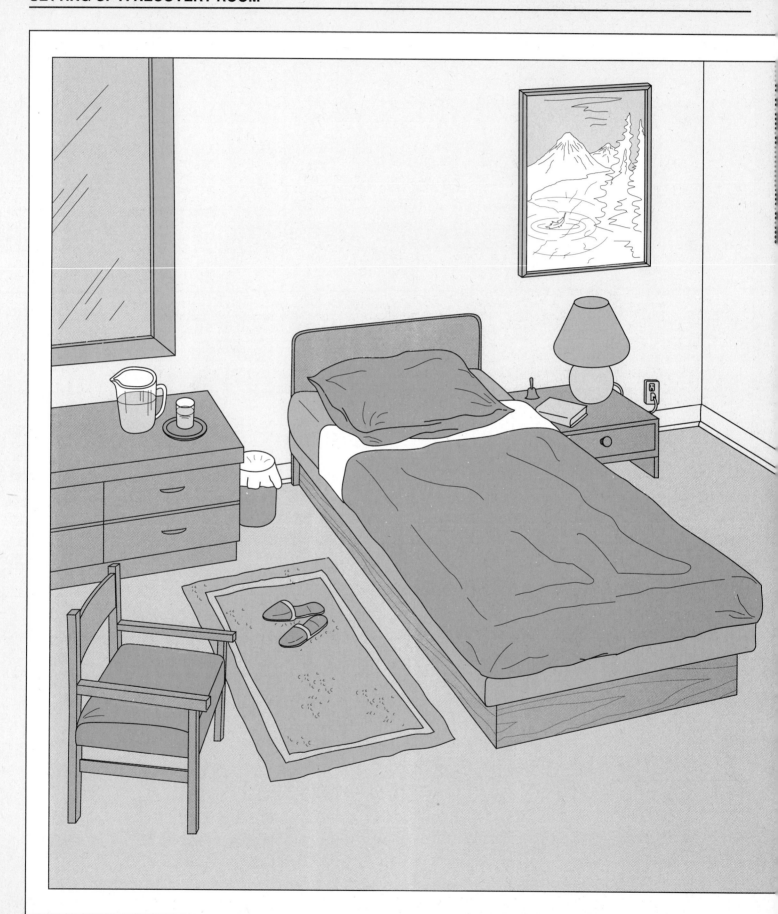

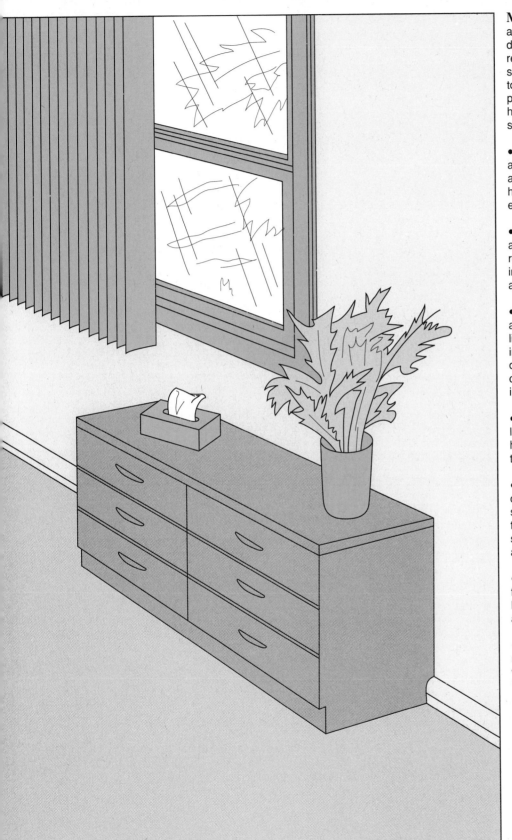

Making a patient comfortable. A pleasant, comfortable environment can make a difference for a family member who is ill or recuperating from an illness. By boosting the spirit and disposition of a patient, you can help to ensure that his recovery is as speedy as possible—and help to minimize the ordeal of his illness. Use the guidelines listed below in setting up a recovery room for a patient:

• Choose a recovery room for a patient in a location that can be kept private and quiet, away from the flow of traffic through your home, but near a bathroom and within easy earshot of other rooms in the house.

• Ensure that the recovery room is ventilated adequately, but is not drafty. If the air of the room tends to be dry, set up a humidifier to increase humidity. **Caution:** Never position a humidifier where a child can grab or tip it.

• Position a bed for the patient in a spot near a window that maximizes the benefits of sunlight, allowing natural warmth and brightness into the room. Make sure that window blinds or shades are adjusted to prevent glare and can be closed to block out sunlight completely in the event that the patient needs sleep.

• Make up the bed for the patient with fresh linen, keeping extra pillows and blankets on hand nearby. Provide the patient with clean towels and facecloths for only his use.

• Furnish the recovery room with a chest of drawers for clothing, a bedside table for personal items and a comfortable armchair; position them within easy reach of the bed. Make sure that the floor is kept free of obstacles; any rug should be slip-proof.

• Cheer the atmosphere of the room with flowers and pictures, without adding clutter. Keep the room clean, tidy and free of unpleasant odors.

• Provide the patient with a bright light for reading; if necessary, also a night light. Place within reach of the patient a bell for summoning help, a pitcher of fresh water and a drinking glass, a box of tissues, a wastebasket lined with a plastic bag, and personal items such as a hairbrush and hand mirror, a writing pad and pen, and books or magazines.

MONITORING TEMPERATURE

Using a thermometer. Temperature readings of the body are important in diagnosing illnesses. For an adult or child, an oral temperature can usually be taken *(step right)*; take the rectal temperature of an infant *(step below, left)*. A less accurate temperature reading can be taken at the armpit *(step below, right)* if an oral or rectal temperature cannot be taken—when a patient is suffering from recurring bouts of vomiting and diarrhea, for example.

To take a temperature reading, use a thermometer: an oral mercury type for an oral or armpit temperature; a rectal mercury type for a rectal or armpit temperature. (A rectal thermometer is identifiable by its short, round end.) An electronic type of thermometer can be used for an oral, rectal or armpit temperature; it takes less time to provide a temperature reading than a mercury type of thermometer.

Body temperature can fluctuate during the day; typically, it is lowest first thing in the morning, rising through the course of the day. A temperature reading is most reliable if the patient is kept calm and quiet for 20 to 30 minutes prior to the taking of it. Keep in mind that a temperature reading can be affected by factors such as clothing, eating, drinking or smoking, physical activity or emotional stress, and the ambient temperature of the room.

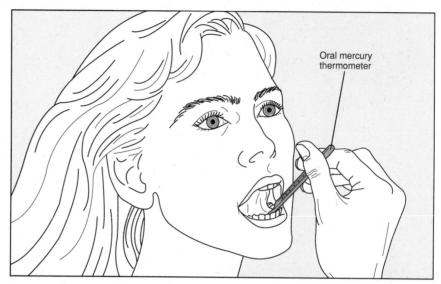

Oral mercury thermometer

Taking an oral temperature. To use an oral mercury thermometer, wipe the bulb using a cotton ball moistened with rubbing alcohol, then rinse it thoroughly in cool water. Hold the thermometer by the end opposite the bulb to shake the mercury below the 95°F mark, flicking your wrist downward. Place the bulb of the thermometer under the tongue *(above)* and close the mouth; hold the thermometer using the lips and not with the teeth. Leave the thermometer in place for at least 2 minutes, then remove it to take a reading. To use an electronic thermometer, follow the manufacturer's instructions. A normal oral temperature reading is 98.6°F; a slightly higher reading can be normal for a child. Treat a high or low temperature *(page 115)*.

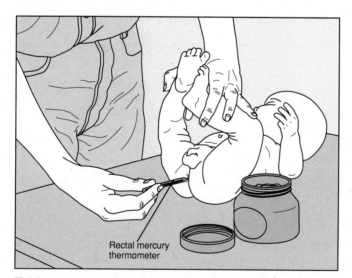

Rectal mercury thermometer

Taking a rectal temperature. To use a rectal mercury thermometer, wipe the bulb using a cotton ball moistened with rubbing alcohol. Hold the thermometer by the end opposite the bulb to shake the mercury below the 95°F mark. For an infant, lie him on his back and hold his legs up by the ankles; for an adult or child, lie him on his side with his legs drawn up. Dip the bulb of the thermometer in petroleum jelly and insert it no more than 1 inch into the rectum *(above)*; hold it in place for 3 to 5 minutes. Remove the thermometer to take a reading. To use an electronic thermometer, follow the manufacturer's instructions. A normal rectal temperature reading is 99.6°F; a slightly higher reading can be normal for an infant or child. Treat a high or low temperature *(page 115)*.

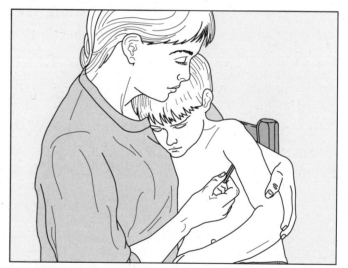

Taking an armpit temperature. To use a mercury thermometer, wipe the bulb using a cotton ball moistened with rubbing alcohol. Hold the thermometer by the end opposite the bulb to shake the mercury below the 95°F mark. Wipe the armpit dry using a clean towel, then place the bulb of the thermometer against the center of it. Holding the thermometer in place, gently press the arm into the armpit and bend it at the elbow to rest it across the chest *(above)*. Leave the thermometer in place for at least 15 minutes, then remove it to take a reading. To use an electronic thermometer, follow the manufacturer's instructions. A normal armpit temperature reading is 97.6°F; a slightly higher reading can be normal for an infant or child. Treat a high or low temperature *(page 115)*.

TREATING A HIGH OR LOW TEMPERATURE

Handling an abnormal temperature reading. An abnormally high body temperature, or fever, is usually due to an infection, but can be caused by a reaction to medication or provoked by a medical emergency such as a heart attack or stroke. An abnormally low body temperature can be caused by a reaction to medication or result from shock or prolonged exposure to extreme cold. An extremely high or low body temperature can be a sign of a medical emergency; immediately seek emergency help for a patient with a temperature above 102°F or below 97°F. Consult your physician about any abnormal temperature of a patient who is less than 12 months of age or very old; is diagnosed with a serious disease or condition; has just started taking a medication; or complains of lethargy, breathing difficulty, earache, neck stiffness or a rash.

A family member typically is far more likely to suffer a fever than a low body temperature. In many instances, however, a fever is not a cause for alarm and can be handled effectively at home. The pattern of a fever can vary, often rising and falling from hour to hour and from day to day. Monitor the temperature *(page 114)* of a family member who is ill or recuperating from an illness every 1 to 2 hours through the course of each day—or at the time interval recommended by your physician. Keep a record of the temperature readings of the patient for reference in the event you must consult your physician; it can help him in his diagnosis.

Take measures to treat the fever of a patient at home as soon as you detect it using the guidelines below:

• Have the patient rest in bed with a minimum of blankets and other bedcovers; have him remove excess clothing.

• Keep the recovery room of the patient cool—about 60° F.

• Provide the patient with cool baths or sponge baths. Administer cool—not cold—compresses to the body areas of the patient where heat is greatest: the head, neck, chest, armpits and groin.

• Have the patient drink plenty of liquids to replenish fluids lost by sweating; he should drink at least 1 1/2 pints of liquid daily.

• Do not try to "sweat out" the fever by overheating the patient.

• If the fever of the patient does not subside within 1 to 2 hours, administer a nonprescription pain-reliever *(page 121)*.

• Consult your physician if the fever is accompanied by other symptoms, or it does not subside in an infant within a few hours, in a child within 24 hours, or in an adult within 48 hours.

MONITORING A PULSE

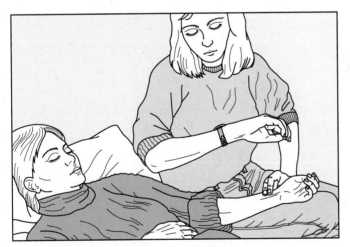

Taking the pulse of an adult or child. Pulse readings can help in identifying the severity of illnesses. Take the pulse of an adult or child at the radial artery. Lie the patient on his back, then place your index and middle fingers on the inside of his wrist just below the thumb; do not use your thumb. Press gently into the wrist of the patient and count his pulse for 30 seconds *(above)*. Obtain the pulse per minute by multiplying your count by 2 and record it. A normal pulse is strong, regular and 60 to 100 beats per minute for an adult; 80 to 100 beats per minute for a child. The pulse of an adult or child who is ill or recuperating from an illness may be higher than normal, especially if he has a fever. If there is no pulse or the pulse is weak or irregular, immediately seek emergency medical help.

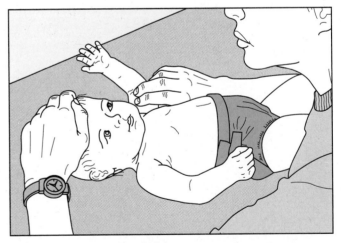

Taking the pulse of an infant. Pulse readings can help in identifying the severity of illnesses. Take the pulse of an infant at the brachial artery. Lie the patient on his back, then place your index and middle fingers on the inside of his upper arm midway between the shoulder and elbow; do not use your thumb. Press gently into the upper arm of the patient and count his pulse for 30 seconds *(above)*. Obtain the pulse per minute by multiplying your count by 2 and record it. A normal pulse for an infant is strong, regular and 100 to 125 beats per minute. The pulse of an infant who is ill or recuperating from an illness may be higher than normal, especially if he has a fever. If there is no pulse or the pulse is weak or irregular, immediately seek emergency medical help.

MOVING A PATIENT

Assisting a bedridden patient. A family member who is ill or recuperating from an illness may need assistance to turn over in bed *(step below)*, sit up in bed or get out of bed *(page 117)*. If possible, encourage and help a patient to get out of bed for at least part of the day—even if only to sit for a short while in a chair. Provide the patient with assistance in moving using good body mechanics; follow the guidelines listed below:

• If possible, have a helper assist you in moving the patient—especially if he is obese. Do not attempt to move a patient alone if you cannot handle his weight or you suffer from a back problem or other disabling injury or condition.

• Wear comfortable, low-heeled shoes with non-slip soles and closed backs to move the patient.

• Keep as close to the patient as possible to move him. Stand with your back straight, your feet apart by about the width of your shoulders and your knees bent slightly; this position provides you with stable footing and as much of a support base as possible.

• Support the patient using the muscles of your legs and arms—not your back. Bend down at your knees, keeping your back straight. Do not bend or twist at the waist.

• Have the patient cooperate in providing you with as much self-support as he can.

A patient who is confined to bed for an extended period of time can develop bedsores, painful ulcerations of the skin that reduce the circulation of blood and lead to damage of the skin tissue. The areas of the body most prone to bedsores include the elbows, the heels and the back at the base of the spine. For a patient who is confined to bed and cannot get up to move around, you can help to prevent bedsores by following the guidelines listed below:

• Keep the bed linen and clothes of the patient clean, dry and smooth. Tuck the sheets tightly to prevent them wrinkling.

• Change the position of the patient every 2 to 3 hours during the day, if possible. Assist the patient to turn over *(step below)* or sit up *(page 117)* in bed; avoid dragging him.

• Encourage the patient to establish periods of exercise—wriggling the toes and fingers, rotating the ankles and wrists, flexing the muscles of the arms and legs, and stretching the body, for example.

• Regularly bathe the patient in bed *(page 118)*, patting him dry thoroughly with a towel; pay close attention to the folds of his skin.

• Apply a skin oil product and massage the patient, focusing on the areas of his body that bear his weight in bed.

• Keep pillows between the ankles of the patient to prevent them from rubbing together.

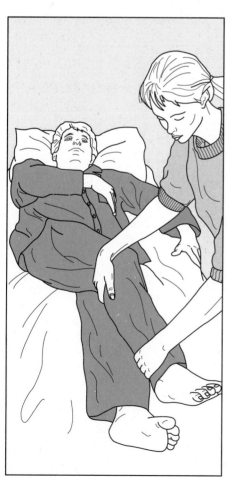
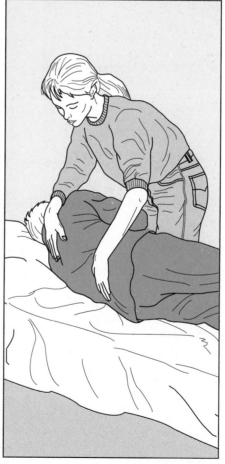

Turning a patient over in bed. Positioning yourself to face the front of the patient as you turn him, stand on one side of the bed with one foot slightly in front of the other foot. Place the arm of the patient closest to you along his side and the other arm across his chest, bending it at the elbow. Cross the legs of the patient at the ankles, bending the leg farthest from you at the knee and hip to bring it over the other leg *(far left)*. Reaching across the patient, use one hand to grip his shoulder securely and slide the other hand under his lower back. Shifting your weight from your front foot to your back foot, roll the patient toward you in one smooth motion, shifting your hand on his shoulder to the base of his neck *(near left)*. To keep the patient on his side, straighten his lower leg, then bend his upper leg at the knee and hip to cross it. If necessary, use pillows to support the upper leg of the patient.

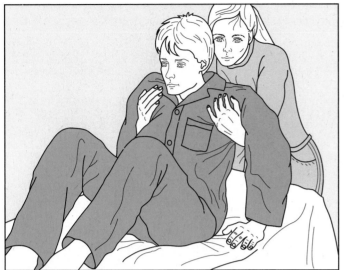

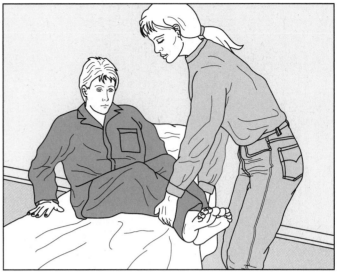

Sitting a patient up in bed. Stand behind the patient at the head of the bed; if necessary, move it out from the wall to reach him. Have the patient draw his legs up toward his chest, bending them at the knees and hips, then plant the soles of his feet flat on the bed. Slide your arms under and around the shoulders of the patient, grasping him securely. Having the patient push downward with his hands and feet, bend down at your knees and stand straight up, lifting his upper body *(above, left)*; keep your back straight. If necessary, help the patient to position himself comfortably with pillows. To assist the patient in sitting at the edge of the bed, move to his feet and grasp them securely just above the ankles. Having the patient push downward with his hands, lift his legs and swing them off the edge of the bed *(above, right)*, helping him to pivot at the waist.

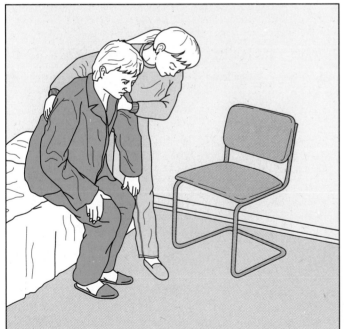

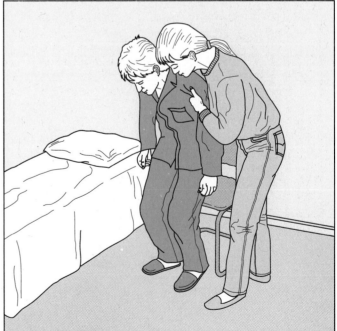

Getting a patient out of bed. Assist the patient in sitting up at the edge of the bed *(step above)*; if necessary, help him put on slippers. Have the patient push downward with his hands to move himself as close to the edge of the bed as possible; stand facing him and lean slightly toward him to keep him from falling off it. Then, position yourself on one side of the patient with one foot slightly ahead of the other foot. Grasp the patient securely under the shoulders; if necessary, drape his arm closest to you across your shoulder to give him added support. Shifting your weight from your front foot to your back foot, bend down at your knees and stand straight up, lifting his upper body to help him stand *(above, left)*; keep your back straight. Give the patient time to adjust to standing, then have him lean against you and slowly move forward, taking short, smooth steps and following his pace. When you reach your destination, help the patient to sit *(above, right)* and position himself comfortably.

BATHING A PATIENT IN BED

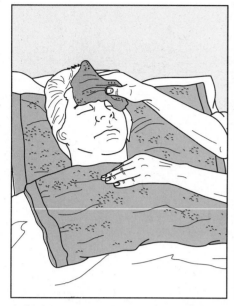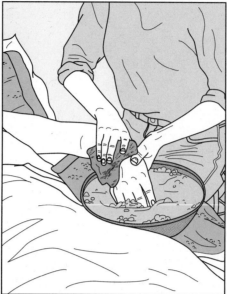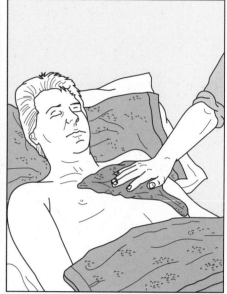

1 **Bathing the face, arms and chest.** A family member who is ill or recuperating from an illness may be unable to take a bath or shower. To bathe the patient in bed, have him remove his clothing, then cover him with a sheet to keep him warm. Fill a basin with warm water and have on hand a supply of clean facecloths and bath towels; if using soap, also another basin of warm water for rinsing. Soak a facecloth in the water and wring it before wiping the patient with it, starting with his face *(above, left)* and neck; use a towel to keep the bedding dry. If you are washing the patient using soap, rinse his face and neck with water using another facecloth. Dry the face and neck of the patient immediately, patting gently with a towel; avoid any rubbing. Bathe each arm of the patient the same way, dipping his hand into the water *(above, center)*. Continue using the same procedure, uncovering only the part of the patient you are bathing *(above, right)*, then covering it again. Change the water of the basin as soon as it cools or becomes dirty.

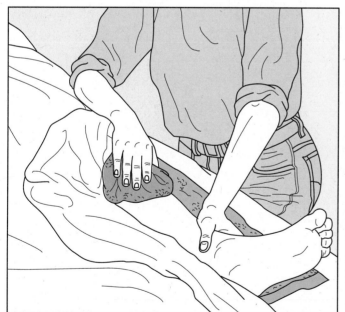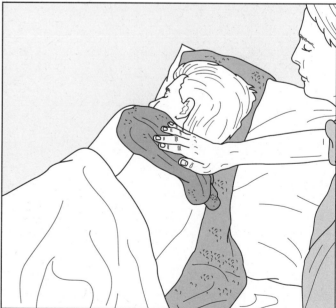

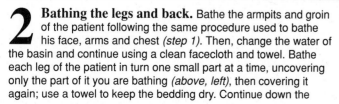

2 **Bathing the legs and back.** Bathe the armpits and groin of the patient following the same procedure used to bathe his face, arms and chest *(step 1)*. Then, change the water of the basin and continue using a clean facecloth and towel. Bathe each leg of the patient in turn one small part at a time, uncovering only the part of it you are bathing *(above, left)*, then covering it again; use a towel to keep the bedding dry. Continue down the front of the patient to his toes the same way, changing the water of the basin as soon as it cools or becomes dirty. If you are washing the patient using soap, be sure that you rinse thoroughly with water using another facecloth. Remember to only pat the patient dry with the towel. Have the patient turn onto his side; if necessary, assist him *(page 116)*. Then, bathe the back *(above, right)*, buttocks and other parts of the patient that you could not reach from his front.

ADMINISTERING HEAT TREATMENTS

Using heat treatments. The application of heat to an area of the body warms it and dilates the blood vessels near its surface, increasing blood circulation. Heat treatments can be used to help relieve everyday tension of muscles, ease chronic stiffness or pain of muscles and joints, or promote the healing of strained or sprained muscles and ligaments 48 hours following an injury.

There are two basic types of heat treatments: dry heat applied with a hot-water bottle, a chemical hot pack or a heating pad *(step right)*; moist heat applied with a hot compress or a hot bath *(step below)*. Moist heat tends to be more effective than dry heat, penetrating warmth deeply into the body. Administer any heat treatment using the guidelines listed below:

• Apply cold treatments *(page 120)* for the first 48 hours following an injury. Heat treatments administered too soon after an injury can re-open a wound, causing added bleeding, and increase swelling, causing added pain.

• Never apply heat treatments to an area of the body with reduced sensation.

• Administer heat treatments for only 15 to 20 minutes at a time. If redness of the skin after a heat treatment does not disappear within a few minutes, wait 3 to 4 hours before continuing with a lower-temperature heat treatment.

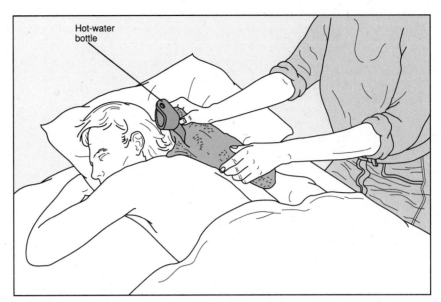

Hot-water bottle

Administering dry heat treatments. Prepare a hot-water bottle with water that is hot—not boiling. Pour the hot water into the hot-water bottle until it is about 2/3 full. Set the hot-water bottle carefully on its side without spilling it, then press gently against it to expel air and screw on its cap tightly. Wrap the hot-water bottle with a towel and apply it to the affected area of the body *(above)*. Remove the hot-water bottle from the affected area of the body after 15 to 20 minutes. Prepare a chemical hot pack by boiling water and removing it from the heat, then immersing the hot pack in it for 7 minutes. Administer the hot pack as you would a hot-water bottle. Use a heating pad following the same guidelines. Wait for at least 1 hour before readministering a heat treatment.

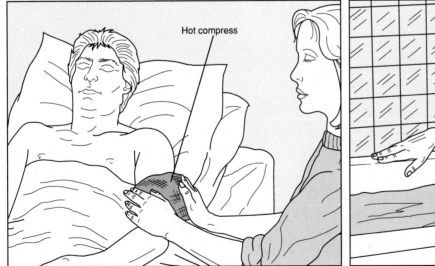

Hot compress

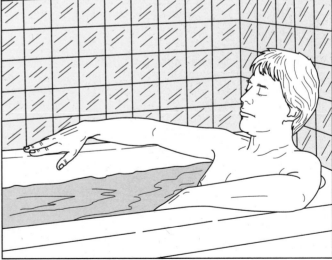

Administering moist heat treatments. Prepare a hot compress by boiling water, then let it cool until it is comfortable to the touch. Soak a facecloth and a towel in the hot water and wring them thoroughly. Fold the facecloth into a pad slightly larger than the affected area of the body, then cover it with plastic kitchen wrap to help it retain heat and wrap the towel around it. Apply the hot compress to the affected area of the body *(above, left)*; when it cools, reheat the towel with hot water. Continue the same way for 15 to 20 minutes. Prepare a hot bath with water as hot as can be tolerated; if desired, add a little sea salt. Soak the body in the hot bath *(above, right)* for 15 to 20 minutes. Wait for at least 1 hour before readministering a heat treatment.

ADMINISTERING COLD TREATMENTS

Using cold treatments. The application of cold to an area of the body cools it and constricts the blood vessels near its surface, decreasing blood circulation. Cold treatments can be used to help stop the flow of blood from a wound or 48 hours after an injury occurs to help reduce its swelling, inflammation and pain, as well as promote its healing.

There are two basic types of cold treatments: dry cold applied with an ice pack or a chemical cold pack *(step right)*; moist cold applied with a cold compress, a cold bath or a cold-mist humidifier *(step below)*. Dry cold tends to be more effective than moist cold; it can be tolerated by an area of the body at a temperature low enough to help numb any pain. Administer any cold treatment using the guidelines listed below:

• Apply heat treatments *(page 119)* after the first 48 hours following an injury. Cold treatments administered too late after an injury can slow healing—without reducing pain.

• Never apply cold treatments to any area of the body with reduced sensation.

• Administer cold treatments for only 15 to 20 minutes at a time. If sensitivity of the skin does not return within a few minutes after a cold treatment, wait 2 to 3 hours before continuing with a higher-temperature cold treatment.

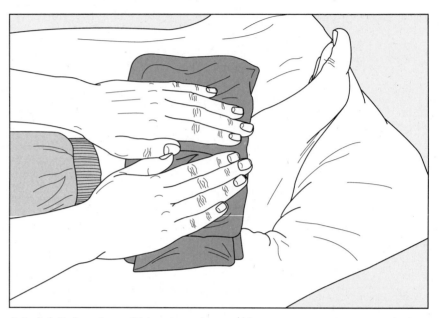

Administering dry cold treatments. Prepare an ice pack using crushed ice. Fill a plastic bag with ice cubes and wrap it with a towel, then crush the ice cubes using a rolling pin or a hammer. Pour the crushed ice into the ice pack until it is about half full, then screw on its cap tightly. Wrap the ice pack with a towel and apply it to the affected area of the body *(above)*. Remove the ice-pack from the affected area of the body after 15 to 20 minutes. Prepare a chemical ice pack by placing it in the freezer for at least 2 hours, then administer it the same way. Wait for at least 1 hour before readministering a cold treatment.

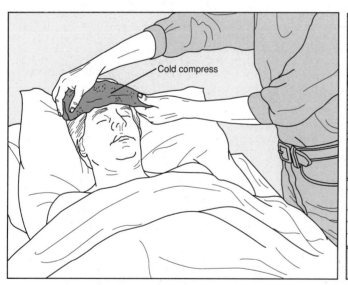

Cold compress

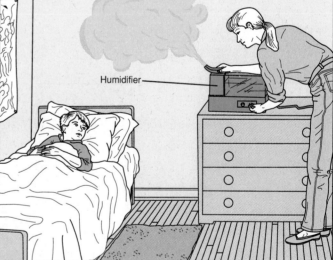

Humidifier

Administering moist cold treatments. Prepare a cold compress using ice water, filling a bowl with ice cubes and cold water. Soak a facecloth and a towel in the ice water and wring them thoroughly. Fold the facecloth into a pad slightly larger than the affected area of the body, then cover it with plastic kitchen wrap to help it retain cold and wrap the towel around it. Apply the cold compress to the affected area of the body *(above, left)*; when it warms, re-cool the towel with ice water. Continue the same way for 15 to 20 minutes. Prepare a cold bath with water as cold as can be tolerated, then soak the affected area of the body in it for 15 to 20 minutes. Wait for at least 30 minutes before readministering a cold compress or a cold bath. To relieve nasal congestion, set up a cold-mist humidifier *(above, right)* following the manufacturer's instructions.

ADMINISTERING NONPRESCRIPTION PAIN-RELIEVERS

Using nonprescription pain-relievers. To help ease the suffering of a minor ache or pain, a family member may need to use a nonprescription pain-reliever. A nonprescription pain-reliever acts to ease an ache or pain at the site of its origin—unlike a prescription pain-reliever that acts to ease an ache or pain at the level of the central nervous system. A nonprescription pain-reliever does not eliminate the cause of an ache or pain, but can suppress it to a level that is tolerable; acetaminophen and aspirin types also help to bring down fever.

Before resorting to the use of a nonprescription pain-reliever, try alternative pain remedies such as hot *(page 119)* or cold *(page 120)* treatments and relaxation techniques. If the use of a nonprescription pain-reliever is necessary, choose an acetaminophen or aspirin type; although ibuprofen types can be purchased without a prescription, their use is recommended only for adults under the close supervision of a physician. **Caution:** Aspirin is not recommended for children under the age of 15 due to its link with the incidence of Reye's Syndrome.

• Always administer nonprescription pain-relievers following the recommended dosages—typically given in milligrams (mg). Never take more of a nonprescription pain-reliever than recommended within a time period.

• Avoid decisions on nonprescription pain-relievers based on hasty comparisons between extra-strength types and regular-strength types; extra-strength types are usually more expensive, but simply contain more ingredient per tablet or capsule—which can make dosage more difficult to regulate.

• Sensitivity to nonprescription pain-relievers can vary depending on the type and the individual. Skin rashes and asthmatic-like shortness of breath are common signs of a possible allergy. Discontinue use of a nonprescription pain-reliever the moment you detect any side effects; report the side effects to your physician.

Always read the label carefully before purchasing or administering a nonprescription pain-reliever *(page 122)*. Follow the manufacturer's instructions for the usage of a nonprescription pain-reliever to the letter; also pay close attention to information on warnings and possible side effects. Check with your physician before using a nonprescription pain-reliever if you are taking another medication or you are pregnant. Consult your physician before administering a nonprescription pain-reliever to an infant under 12 months of age.

Refer to the chart below for guidelines on the use of nonprescription pain-relievers; the common types included are sold under a variety of trade names and are readily available at your local pharmacy. Do not hesitate to ask your physician or pharmacist for help in choosing a nonprescription pain-reliever—or any questions about the administering of a particular type. Use a nonprescription pain-reliever cautiously; its availability without a prescription does not make it less potentially harmful than other medication. Observe the following precautions:

• Stomach upset is a common problem associated with the taking of nonprescription pain-relievers, especially aspirin types; acetaminophen types are less likely to cause stomach upset. To help minimize stomach upset, take any nonprescription pain-reliever with a glass of water shortly after eating a meal.

• Taking the maximum recommended dosage of a nonprescription pain-reliever can risk the provoking of toxic effects: sweating, dizziness, headache, nausea or vomiting, drowsiness or confusion, or fever. At the first sign of these symptoms, immediately consult your physician.

• Never administer a nonprescription pain-reliever for an extended time period. Limit the number of consecutive days a nonprescription pain-reliever is taken: 5 days for an adult; 3 days for a child. If an ache, pain or other problem persists, consult your physician.

TYPE OF MEDICATION	PURPOSE	RECOMMENDED DOSAGE	POSSIBLE SIDE EFFECTS
Acetaminophen	For relief of minor ache or pain, fever (especially of a child), or headache; recommended for patient with allergy or sensitivity to aspirin	Adult: Usually 325 mg to 650 mg (1 to 2 tablets or capsules) every 3 to 4 hours up to 8 times a day Child over 10: Usually 600 mg every 4 to 6 hours up to 6 times a day Child up to 10: Usually 60 mg per year of age every 4 to 6 hours up to 6 times a day	Diarrhea Sweating Appetite loss Nausea or vomiting Stomach cramps Abdominal or stomach tenderness, swelling or pain
Aspirin (Buffered or enteric-coated type reduces risk of stomach upset)	For relief of minor ache or pain, fever, toothache, or headache	Adult: Usually 325 mg to 650 mg (1 to 2 tablets or capsules) every 3 to 4 hours up to 8 times a day Child over 15: Usually 600 mg every 4 to 6 hours up to 6 times a day Child up to 15: Not recommended	Nausea or vomiting Heartburn Allergic reaction Ear ringing Headache Dizziness Breathing rapidity Irritability
Ibuprofen	For relief of inflammation, swelling, stiffness or pain under supervision of physician	Adult: Usually 200 mg (1 tablet) every 4 to 6 hours up to 6 times a day Child: Not recommended	Nausea Diarrhea Dizziness

USING MEDICATION

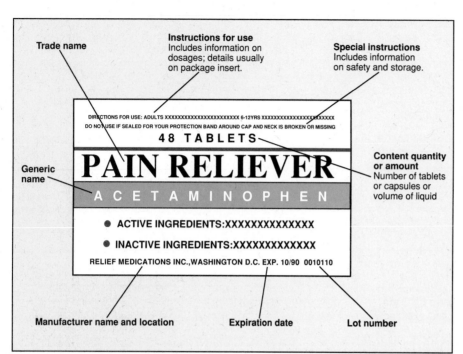

Trade name

Instructions for use
Includes information on dosages; details usually on package insert.

Special instructions
Includes information on safety and storage.

DIRECTIONS FOR USE: ADULTS XXXXXXXXXXXXXXXXXXXXXXX 6-12YRS XXXXXXXXXXXXXXXXXXXXXXXX
DO NOT USE IF SEALED FOR YOUR PROTECTION BAND AROUND CAP AND NECK IS BROKEN OR MISSING

48 TABLETS

PAIN RELIEVER
ACETAMINOPHEN

Generic name

Content quantity or amount
Number of tablets or capsules or volume of liquid

● ACTIVE INGREDIENTS:XXXXXXXXXXXXXX

● INACTIVE INGREDIENTS:XXXXXXXXXXXXX

RELIEF MEDICATIONS INC.,WASHINGTON D.C. EXP. 10/90 0010110

Manufacturer name and location

Expiration date

Lot number

Reading a medication label. As a rule, you should avoid the use of any medication unless it is recommended by your physician. When you must use a medication, always read and follow the information on its label carefully. Illustrated at left is the label of a typical nonprescription pain-reliever; refer to it for the various types of information you should know about a medication.

Although a medication may be considered as safe if it is taken strictly following the manufacturer's instructions, it should always be used cautiously. When you require a medication, do not hesitate to ask your physician or pharmacist for guidance in choosing the type best suited to your particular medical problem or condition. For specific details on a medication, write to its manufacturer.

Using medication safely. A medication can cause unintended harm far surpassing its intended benefit if it is not used properly. Always use any medication cautiously, following the precautions listed below:

● Before administering a medication, carefully read the information provided on its label *(step above)* and any package insert.

● Consult your physician before administering a nonprescription medication to an infant.

● Be sure that you administer a medication in accordance with its format: by medicine dropper or spoon; by diluting or dissolving; by ingesting with water; by inhaling; by applying directly to the skin.

● Administer only the specified amount of a medication at only the specified times. Never administer a prescription medication to other than the patient for whom it is prescribed.

● Be alert to the possible side effects of a medication; discontinue use of the medication if any side effects are detected and report them to your physician.

● Store medication out of the reach of children. Always put a medication away as soon as you have finished administering it; never leave it out and unattended.

● Discard leftover medication and any medication beyond its expiration date.

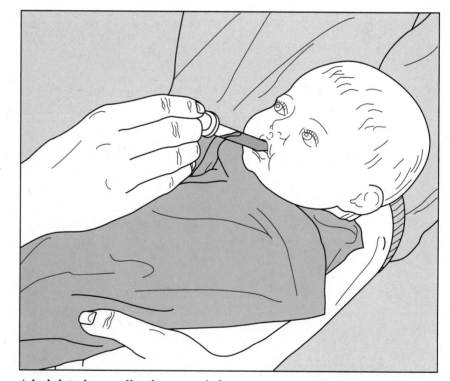

Administering medication to an infant. Medication for an infant is usually provided in liquid form. To administer the medication, wash your hands thoroughly with soap and water. Using a sterile calibrated medicine dropper, squeeze the bulb and insert the tip of the tube into the medication. Slowly release pressure on the bulb, drawing the correct dosage of the medication into the tube. Gently insert the tip of the tube into the mouth of the infant *(above)* and squeeze the bulb to slowly release the medication. For an older infant, you may pour the correct dosage of the medication into a sterile calibrated medicine spoon, then administer it the same way.

CHANGING BANDAGES

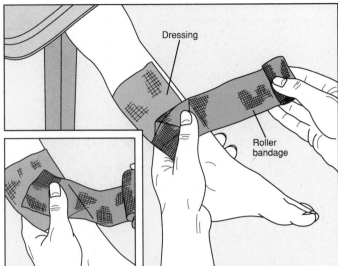

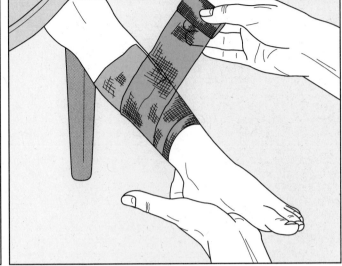

Rebandaging a leg or arm. Gently remove the old bandage and dressing from the wound. Carefully wash the wound with soap and water, then pat it dry with a clean towel. Cover the wound with a sterile gauze dressing and secure it in place with a narrow gauze roller bandage—tight enough to hold it without restricting blood circulation. Starting at the narrowest part of the limb on one side of the dressing, wrap the roller bandage once around the limb, allowing one corner of it to protrude *(inset)*. Fold the corner over the first turn, then secure it by wrapping the roller bandage around the limb *(above, left)* and over it. Continue wrapping the roller bandage around the limb until the dressing is covered, overlapping it by 1/3 to 1/2 its width each turn *(above, right)*. Wrap the roller bandage around the limb several extra turns, then hold it in place and use scissors to snip off the excess. Secure the end of the roller bandage using medical tape or a safety pin; or, snip it along the center, then wrap the strands in opposite directions and tie them together.

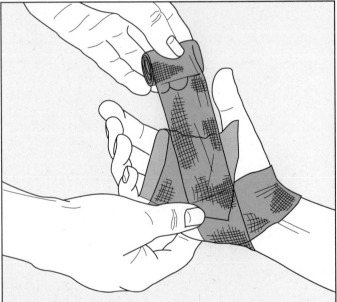

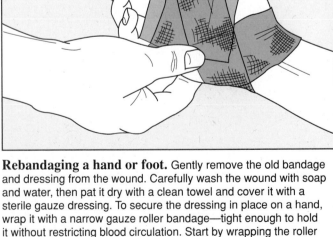

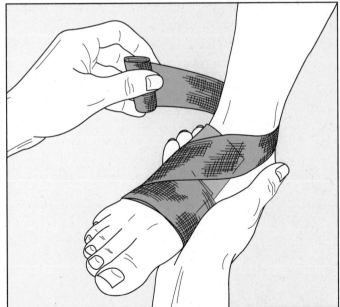

Rebandaging a hand or foot. Gently remove the old bandage and dressing from the wound. Carefully wash the wound with soap and water, then pat it dry with a clean towel and cover it with a sterile gauze dressing. To secure the dressing in place on a hand, wrap it with a narrow gauze roller bandage—tight enough to hold it without restricting blood circulation. Start by wrapping the roller bandage several turns around the hand, then across it and around the wrist. Cross the roller bandage over the turn around the wrist *(above, left)* and wrap it again around the hand, completing a figure-8 pattern. Continue wrapping the roller bandage around the hand and wrist following the same pattern until the dressing is held in place on the wound, then wrap it several extra turns around the wrist. To secure the dressing in place on a foot, use the same procedure to wrap a roller bandage around the foot and ankle in a figure-8 pattern *(above, right)*. Use scissors to snip off the excess roller bandage, then secure the end of it with medical tape or a safety pin; or, snip it along the center, then wrap the strands in opposite directions and tie them together.

MONITORING YOUR HEALTH

Getting medical checkups. Monitoring your health today can mean striking a reasonable balance between the expense of undergoing full head-to-toe examinations annually and the risks of consulting a physician only once a medical problem develops. If you are in good health, you are not likely to require extensive medical testing every year; depending on personal factors such as family medical history, age and lifestyle, however, selective, periodic physical examinations are prudent and economical.

The first step in monitoring your health is establishing an on-going relationship with your own physician *(page 125)*, following his recommendations for regular checkups. You can expect a basic schedule of regular checkups for yourself that includes the common types of medical tests listed in the chart below, varying according to your personal factors. Regular checkups are critical to maintaining your health: preventing medical problems from occurring; permitting early diagnosis and treatment of any medical problem that does occur.

Depending on your family medical history, your physician may also schedule blood tests and urine tests, routine procedures for the early detection of disorders such as high blood pressure, diabetes, heart disease, kidney disease or cancer. Special tests involving X rays or ultrasound, for example, may be requested by your physician to confirm and supplement his diagnosis using other procedures. In addition, your physician may ask for periodic repeats of certain types of tests as a way to document your personal patterns and monitor changes.

The type and frequency of your checkups should be modified with age and changes in your lifestyle. For example, a rectal examination may not be necessary until the age of 20, then only every 3 to 5 years until the age of 40; from the age of 40, however, it is recommended annually along with a stool test. Or, if a job change means working an a noisy environment, regular hearing tests may be advised.

Ask your physician for guidance on proper self-examination techniques, especially for the breasts or testicles *(page 84)* and blood pressure *(page 56)*. Between regular checkups, consult your physician about any sign of a potentially-serious medical problem; for example:

- A change in bowel or bladder habits
- A sore that does not heal
- Unusual bleeding or discharge
- A lump or thickening under the skin
- Abdominal pain or persisting indigestion
- A change in a wart or mole
- A nagging cough or persisting hoarseness

MEDICAL TEST	PURPOSE	RECOMMENDED FREQUENCY
General physical checkup	For detecting problem with heart, lung or other vital organ	Every 3 to 5 years from age of 20 to age of 40 and annually from age of 40 or as recommended by physician
Eye examination	For detecting problem with vision	Every 3 to 5 years from childhood or as recommended by physician; annually from age of 40 if have family history of glaucoma
Dental checkup	For detecting problem with teeth, gums or mouth	Every 6 to 8 months from childhood to age of 20 and annually from age of 20 or as recommended by dentist
Blood pressure monitoring	For detecting problem with heart or arteries, especially if overweight, taking contraceptive pill, or have family history of high blood pressure, heart or kidney disease, stroke, or diabetes	Every 3 to 5 years from age of 20 or as recommended by physician; annually from age of 20 if overweight or have family history of high blood pressure, heart or kidney disease, stroke, or diabetes; annually if taking contraceptive pill
Serum cholesterol, triglyceride and HDL level tests	For detecting risk of problem with heart or arteries, especially if overweight or have family history of high blood pressure, heart or kidney disease, stroke or diabetes	Once at age of 20 to 25 with follow-up as recommended by physician; every 2 to 3 years from age of 40 to age of 50 and annually from age of 50
Rectal examination	For detecting cancer of rectum, colon or prostate, especially if have family history of colorectal or prostate cancer	Every 3 to 5 years from age of 20 or as recommended by physician; annually (with stool test) from age of 40
Vaginal examination	For detecting problem with pelvic floor, perineum or pelvic organ, especially if pregnant or starting new contraceptive	As recommended by physician
Cervical (Pap) smear	For detecting problem with cervix, especially if periods irregular or bleeding occurs between periods	Annually from start of sexual activity or age of 25 or as recommended by physician
Mammography	For detecting cancer of breast, especially if have family history of breast cancer	Once at age of 35 to 40; follow-up every 2 to 3 years from age of 40 or as recommended by physician

ESTABLISHING A PATIENT-PHYSICIAN RELATIONSHIP

Communicating with your physician. Having your own physician is an important element in maintaining your health and assuring yourself of the best health care in the event of a medical problem. Establishing an on-going relationship with a physician ensures that your full medical history is on record in one place, for reference on a monitoring basis and in an emergency situation. Consider your medical needs and personal preferences when choosing a physician; your confidence and comfort are keys to establishing a successful relationship.

To check the credentials of a physician, you can consult The American Medical Directory; do not ignore your biases for a physician of a particular sex or age, or with an association to a particular hospital. In your research on finding a physician, include questions about office location and hours, emergency service and medical fees. Ask your friends and neighbors for references on physicians. Call around to your local and state medical societies; many of them can provide you with the names of physicians taking new patients in your immediate area.

In establishing an on-going relationship with a physician, you should anticipate a host of detailed questions about your family medical history, your personal medical history and your lifestyle—including your occupation, diet, physical exercise patterns, and consumption of alcohol and cigarettes. With this information, the type and frequency of regular checkups appropriate for you can be planned *(page 124)*, setting in place your personal medical baseline for updating and comparison as dictated by changes in your age and life circumstances.

You can expect your physician to provide you on request with medical information you may need, as well as referrals to medical specialists you may require. Consult your physician about proper techniques for self-examination between regular checkups—asking about the monitoring of your blood pressure *(page 56)* or the checking of your breasts or testicles *(page 84)*, for example. Do not hesitate to inquire about the reasons for procedures and tests your physician performs or requests—or to have an explanation repeated in terms you can understand.

Share your generalized and specific medical concerns with your physician at each consultation; they can be important to the diagnosis and understanding of a medical problem. Keep a medical journal, recording information on any medical problem between consultations with your physician. Be ready to volunteer answers to the questions likely to be asked about a medical problem:

- Is the problem constant?

- In what circumstances does the problem occur or change?

- Is the problem accompanied by other symptoms?

- Does your family have a history of similar problems?

- How long have you suffered from the problem?

- Are you currently taking medication?

ESTABLISHING A MEDICAL COVERAGE STRATEGY

Anticipating your health insurance needs. Annual spending on health care in the United States. is billions of dollars—and still rising. Thanks to advances in medical technology, we live longer than our predecessors; and thanks to our extending life span, advances in medical technology carry a heavier load. For every family, there is a probability of its members needing sophisticated medical treatment at some point in their lives. And with the rise in family expectations for health care comes the rise in family pressure to anticipate its costs.

Every family should establish a strategy for ensuring adequate medical coverage—before the need for it arises. A routine medical checkup or test can lead to financial hardship for a family that does not plan in advance for it. Refer to the information presented at right for common options in the various types of medical coverage that are available. The specific items of the medical coverage obtained by a family should vary according to factors such as its size and income, as well as the age, lifestyle and current health status of its members.

Periodically, every family should also revisit an established strategy for ensuring adequate medical coverage—to keep it updated. The specific items of the medical coverage held by a family need to keep pace with the changes in the factors for initially obtaining them. For example, a family that is planning additional members may need to investigate coverage for childbirth and pediatrics. The same family later may need coverage for a chronic disease such as diabetes; and still later may require coverage for nursing-home care.

- **Fee-for-service.** With this type of plan, as its name implies, there is a fee charged to a family member for each medical service provided. The advantage of this type of plan is its flexibility, allowing a family member to choose his provider of a medical service—a particular physician, a certain specialist or a specific hospital, for example. The disadvantage of this type of plan is its cost; for most families, it is too expensive to be practical.

- **Health maintenance organization (HMO).** With this type of plan, a family member can be provided with a range of medical services by an affiliated group of physicians and other health care professionals for a fixed fee. The advantage of this type of plan is its limited and predictable expense, permitting a family member a degree of control over the costs of medical services he obtains. The disadvantage of this type of plan is its inflexibility; medical services provided to a family member at other than a HMO-affiliated facility are not covered.

- **Preferred provider organization (PPO).** With this type of plan, a family member can combine advantageous elements of the fee-for-service plan and the HMO plan. A family member can be provided with a range of medical services at preset rates by PPO-affiliated physicians and health care professionals or can obtain medical services at added expense at other than a PPO-affiliated facility. With this type of plan, a family member is allowed some degree of choice in his provider of medical services and some degree of control over the costs of medical services he obtains.

INDEX

Page references in *italics* indicate an illustration of the subject mentioned. Page references in **bold** indicate a Troubleshooting Guide for the subject mentioned. A **✛** indicates a condition requiring immediate medical attention.

ACKNOWLEDGMENTS

The editors wish to thank the following:
Bonnie Aikman, Food and Drug Administration, Washington, D.C.; American Association of Poison Control Centers, Washington, D.C.; American Foundation for the Prevention of Venereal Disease, Inc., New York, N.Y.; Judith Asher, Montreal, Que.; Biological Rescue Products, Pottstown, Pa.; Blue Cross and Blue Shield Association, Chicago, Ill.; Beverly Boyarsky, Associate, American Lung Association® The Christmas Seal People®, New York, N.Y.; The Canadian Red Cross Society, Ottawa, Ont.; Equipement de securité Safety Supply, St. Laurent, Que.; Thomas G. Glass, Jr. M.D., F.A.C.S., Clinical Professor of Surgery, University of Texas Health Science Center, San Antonio, Tex.; Carrie Goldig-Rappaport, R.N., Montreal, Que.; Health Insurance Association of America, Washington, D.C.; Velda Lulic, Physiotherapist, Montreal, Que.; Marshall Electronics, Lincolnshire, Ill.; Medic Alert Foundation International, Turlock, Ca.; National Safety Council, Chicago, Ill.; New York City Department of Transportation, Safety Education Unit, New York, N.Y.; Nicolas Pelland, Blainville, Que.; Physical Education Digest, Sudbury, Ont.; Dr. Earl Schwartz, Bowman Gray School of Medicine, Winston-Salem, N.C.; Dr. Brian Ticoll, M.D., Montreal, Que.; Dr. Imelda Toledo, M.D., Chihuahua, Mexico; Theodore G. Tong, Pharm.D., University of Arizona, Tucson, Ariz.

The following persons also assisted in the preparation of this book:
Normand Boudreault, Mitchell Glance, Shirley Grynspan, Jennifer Meltzer, Nicolas Moumouris, Robert Paquet, Shirley Sylvain, Dianne Thomas